Well-Being for the Elderly

Well-Being for the Elderly

Primary Preventive Strategies

Thomas T. H. Wan
Medical College of Virginia
Virginia Commonwealth University

Lexington Books
D.C. Heath and Company/Lexington, Massachusetts/Toronto

Library of Congress Cataloging in Publication Data

Wan, Thomas T. H.
  Well-being for the elderly.

  Bibliography: p.
  Includes index.
  1. Aged—United States—Social conditions—Longitudinal
studies. 2. Social status. 3. Aged—United States—Care
and hygiene—Longitudinal studies. I. Title.
HQ1064.U5W334   1985   305.2'6'0973   84-48682
ISBN 0-669-09752-7 (alk. paper)

Published simultaneously in Canada
Printed in the United States of America on acid-free paper
International Standard Book Number: 0-669-09752-7
Library of Congress Catalog Card Number: 84-48682

To Sylvia, George, and William

Contents

Figures and Tables   ix

Acknowledgments   xiii

1. Introduction   1

Gerontological Health: Its Components and Determinants   3
A Model of Continuity of Social and Physical Well-Being in
    Later Life   3

2. Retirement Patterns   7

Related Research   7
Methodology   8
Results   9
Conclusions   15

3. Widowhood   17

Related Research   17
Methodology   18
Results   19
Conclusions   24

**4. Health Consequences of Major Role Losses in
    Later Life**   27

Related Research   28
Methodology   31
Results   34
Conclusions   38
Appendix 4A   **45**

**5. Social and Economic Consequences of Major Role Losses
    in Later Life**   49

Related Research   50
Methodology   55

Results   57
Conclusions   67
Appendix 5A   71

6. **Retirement Attitudes of Married Couples in Later Life   75**

Related Research   75
Methodology   77
Results   81
Conclusions   86

7. **Major Role Losses and Social Participation of Older Males   89**

Related Research   90
Methodology   91
Results   94
Conclusions   103

8. **Planning for Health and Social Well-Being of the Elderly: A Targeting Approach   109**

Related Research   109
Methodology   111
Results   112
Conclusions   121

9. **Summary and Conclusions   127**

Annotated Bibliography   131
Retirement and Well-Being for the Elderly   132
Widowhood and Well-Being for the Elderly   154
Retirement, Widowhood, and Well-Being for the Elderly   165
Other Relevant Studies   168

Bibliography   181

Index   185

About the Author   191

Figures and Tables

Figures

1-1   A Measurement Model of Physical Health and Social Well-Being 4

1-2   A Theoretical Model of Gerontological Health and Role Loss 5

4-1   Generic Model for Explaining Poor Physical Health 34

5-1   Generic Model for Explaining Poor Social Well-Being 56

5-2   A Model for Explaining the Structural Relationship between Physical Health and Social Well-Being for Older Adults in Later Life 64

6-1   Hypothetical Model to Estimate the Retirement Attitudes of Married Couples in Later Life 80

8-1   Predictor Trees for Automatic Interaction Detector (AID) Analysis of Health Index in 1977 by Selected Predictors 113

8-2   Predictor Trees for Automatic Interaction Detector (AID) Analysis of Health Index in 1979 by Selected Predictors 115

8-3   Predictor Trees for Automatic Interaction Detector (AID) Analysis of the Social Well-Being (SWB) Index in 1977 by Selected Predictors 117

8-4   Predictor Trees for Automatic Interaction Detector (AID) Analysis of the Social Well-Being (SWB) Index in 1979 by Selected Predictors 118

Tables

2-1 Percentage Distributions of Persons Who Retired before Age 65 and at Retirement Age in Six Waves of the Retirement History Study by Age Cohort in 1969   10

2-2 Logistic Regression of the Conditional Probability of Retirement on Selected Predictors and Prior Retirement Status (Lagged Variable)   11

2-3 Mean Distributions of Selected Social and Health Characteristics of a Panel of Older Adults by Switched Retirement Status (Retired to Nonretired) by Survey Year   13

2-4 Logistic Regression of the Conditional Probability of Switching from Retired to Nonretired Status on Selected Predictors   14

3-1 Proportion and Number of Persons by Widowhood Status in the Survey Years, 1969–1979   20

3-2 Mean (Percentage) Distributions of Selected Well-Being Indicators of Older Males by Widowhood Status and Its Effect   21

3-3 Mean (Percentage) Distributions of Selected Well-Being Indicators of Older Females by Widowhood Status and Its Effect   23

4-1 Percentage Distributions of Persons Who Reported Having a Low Level of Physical Well-Being by Health Indicators and Sex   35

4-2 Standardized LISREL Estimates for the Model of Poor Physical Health of Male Sample   36

4-3 Standardized LISREL Estimates for the Model of Poor Physical Health of Female Sample   39

4A-1 Correlation Coefficients, Means, and Standard Deviations for All Variables in the Model of Physical Health   47

5-1 Selected Social Characteristics of Male and Female Panel Samples in 1975   57

5-2 Percentage Distributions of Persons with a Low Level of Social Well-Being (SWB) by Social, Psychological, and Economic Indicators and Sex   58

5-3 Standardized LISREL Estimates for the Model of Poor Social Well-Being (SWB) of the Male Sample   60

5-4 Standardized LISREL Estimates for the Model of Poor Social Well-Being (SWB) of the Female Sample   62

5-5 Standardized LISREL Estimates for the Model of Physical Health (PH) and Social Well-Being (SWB) of the Male Sample   65

5-6 Standardized LISREL Estimates for the Model of Physical Health (PH) and Social Well-Being (SWB) of the Female Sample   66

5A-1 Correlation Coefficients, Means, and Standard Deviations for All Variables in the Model of Social Well-Being   73

6-1 Percentage Distributions of Attitudes toward Retirement by Retirement Status among Men   82

6-2 Percentage Distributions of Attitudes toward Retirement by Retirement Status among Women   83

6-3 Standardized LISREL Estimates for the Model of Retirement Attitudes of Married Couples   84

7-1 Selected Characteristics of the Study Sample in 1971 by Widowhood and Retirement Status   95

7-2 Proportions of Variance in Informal and Formal Social Participation Explained by Major Role Losses, Concomitant Life Changes, Personal Characteristics, and Previous Social Participation   97

7-3 Summary Statistics from Regression Analysis of Social Participation by Selected Predictors   98

7-4 Adjusted Means of Social Participation by Marital Status (1969 and 1971) and Types of Social Participation in 1971   100

7-5 Adjusted Means of Social Participation by Retirement Status (1969 and 1971) and Types of Social Participation in 1971   101

8-1 Automatic Interaction Detector Analysis of the Relative Contribution of Selected Sociodemographic Variables and Lagged Health and Social Well-Being (SWB) Variables in Explaining Variance in Physical Health   114

8-2 Automatic Interaction Detector Analysis of the Relative Contribution of Selected Sociodemographic Variables and Lagged Health and Social Well-Being (SWB) Variables in Explaining Variance in Social Well-Being   116

8-3 Selected Characteristics of Older Adults in Frailty Status in 1977   120

8-4 Summary Statistics of Multiple Classification Analysis of Physician Contacts Made by the Study Panel in 1978   122

8-5 Summary Statistics of Multiple Classification Analysis of Total Family Income of the Study Panel in 1978   123

Acknowledgments

While the author is grateful to many who contributed to this book, special recognition is given to Dr. Lola M. Irelan, former director of the Longitudinal Retirement History Study in the Division of Retirement and Survivor Studies, Social Security Administration, who conducted the ten-year panel study of a national sample of older adults in the United States. Further, I recognize the grant support made by the AARP Andrus Foundation. I am also grateful to Sage Publications, Inc., for its permission to reprint my two articles previously appearing in *Research on Aging*.

Appreciation must be expressed to David W. Singley and Irma C. Reeder for their assistance in preparing chapters 2 and 3 of this book and to Katherine L. Quigley for her computing and editing assistance. I wish to thank Professor Kenneth F. Ferraro for his technical consultations. Finally, I want to thank Marie Wood, Carroll George, and Valeria Norville for typing the manuscript.

1
Introduction

One of the major concerns in gerontological research is to identify the social and health consequences of critical life-change events. Only when the detrimental effects of role losses experienced in later life have been identified can interventive programs be formulated. Previous studies on life events have concentrated on cross-sectional surveys of psychological and social attributes of young adults. Little has been done, however, by using a longitudinal approach to assess the differential impact of life events on the social and physical well-being of a panel of older adults. Further, scientific effort has yet to be directed toward the development of preventive strategies for the target group in which changes in work status, marital status, and other roles may adversely affect their well-being.

This book addresses several key issues regarding health and role loss. First, what are the health and social characteristics of those experiencing role losses? Second, what are the major consequences of role losses such as retirement and widowhood? Third, what are the specific coping responses of the elderly who have experienced a role loss? Finally, what are the mechanisms for reducing the risk of being adversely affected by the experience of role losses such as widowhood and retirement?

This study is undertaken at a time of increasing concern about the dependency needs of the growing aged population. Loss of the work role through involuntary retirement and/or loss of spouse may adversely affect the health and well-being of the elderly if no adequate coping resources or supportive mechanisms are available to them. Cumulative losses experienced in later life make older adults more vulnerable and dependent on others to maintain their independent functioning. In order to adequately understand and prepare for successful aging, it is imperative to systematically examine role losses and their effects.

While there are voluminous studies of life-change events as stress-inducing factors, there is relatively little known about the long-term impact of role losses on well-being. This lack of knowledge is especially apparent in examining how role losses influence the aging process. This research will further elucidate the magnitude and nature of the role losses most likely to be experienced by the elderly, and how these role losses change their expectations for and perceptions of their lives. In order to determine the cause-effect relationship between role losses and well-being levels of the elderly, careful analysis of panel data is needed.

A life event that results in a role loss might be expected to have a deleterious impact on the well-being of the elderly. Research literature to date has suggested that maladjustment of the elderly in role transitions may be manifested in physical, psychological, or social ways. For example, the role-stress model emphasizes the importance of viewing adjustment to role transitions as a social process [1, 2]. Yet the long-term effects of role transitions on the physical and social well-being of the elderly have not been fully demonstrated. Thus, one cannot be certain that poor physical and social functioning of the elderly are solely attributable to critical life events.

Although a major role loss such as retirement or widowhood does not necessarily exert a significant negative effect on the health of the elderly, evidence has shown that the concurrence of both losses might cause problems of adjustment [3]. Research that deals with the timing of role losses may shed some light on their effects.

The present study will focus on a number of aspects of the aging process. Based upon repeated measurements of work, socioeconomic status, and health status at several points in time, the ten-year Longitudinal Retirement History Survey (LRHS) provides a panel data set that permits the causal ordering of events concerning multiple role losses and their relationships to the level of well-being of the elderly. The causal specification can clarify the direction for program intervention. For example, if role loss does have a deleterious effect on the elderly, a supportive mechanism may be formulated. Second, previous studies have reported the short-term impact of the life-change event, but its long-term impact has yet to be explored in a longitudinal study design. The analysis of multiple waves of panel data provides valuable information about the correlates of retirement and is presented in chapter 2. The differential patterns of widowhood are presented in chapter 3. Further, the well-being of the target groups is examined in multidimensional aspects of physical, psychological, and socioeconomic statuses; therefore, a comprehensive intervention program can be suggested from the analysis of the health and social consequences of role losses in later years.

Gerontological Health: Its Components and Determinants

The general well-being of the elderly can be portrayed by both objectively and subjectively assessed health indicators [4]. Assessment of physical health in terms of an elderly person's functional capacities, presence of chronic conditions, and perceptions of health is especially important in determining the need for health services required in later life. Similarly, analysis of social, economic, and psychological well-being of the elderly may show the need for income maintenance, social adaptation, and planning for the life transition.

The construct of health or well-being is a multidimensional concept which can be operationally measured by physical health, psychological, and social indicators. In order to facilitate the development of social planning strategies, the present study has formulated a measurement model specifying two distinct but related concepts, labeled as physical health and social well-being. Each concept is treated as an underlying construct (latent variable) of health and can be measured by observable indicators (see figure 1-1). The construct validity of the measurement model for each of the well-being dimensions is explored in chapters 4 and 5. The structural relationship between physical health and social well-being is examined in chapter 5. Furthermore, the social and health profiles of those who experienced poor health or negative social well-being are presented. The identification of the conditioning variables or determinants of health has some practical implications for planning. It addresses questions pertaining to the factors affecting changes in well-being levels, the types of services needed, priorities of social and health interventions, and the kind of population which should be targeted for preretirement education or personal counseling.

A Model of Continuity of Social and Physical Well-Being in Later Life

The four phases of the adaptive process outlined in figure 1-2 are (1) the preconditioned phase, (2) the role transitional phase, (3) the coping or adjustment phase, and (4) the outcome phase. When personal resources are limited and prior levels of health and well-being are relatively weak, individuals might be more vulnerable to the adverse effects of role losses. The identification of conditions which render individuals highly susceptible to critical life events is our primary goal in studying the first

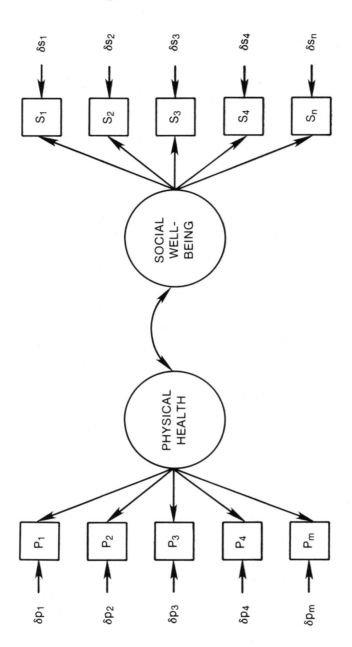

Notes:
 Correlated underlying constructs
P Observable indicator of physical health
S Observable indicator of social well-being
δ Residual error for observable indicator

Figure 1–1. A Measurement Model of Physical Health and Social Well-Being

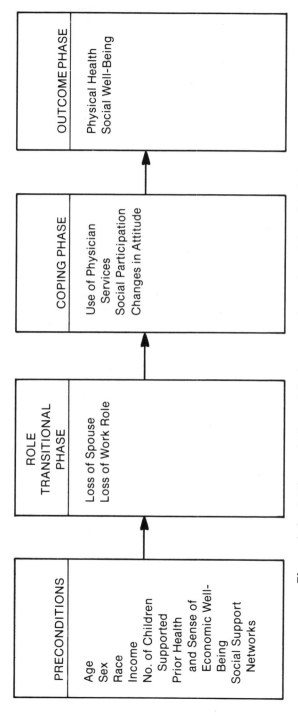

Figure 1–2. A Theoretical Model of Gerontological Health and Role Loss

phase in the social adaptation of the aged. This will serve as a foundation for developing preventive strategies. In the role transitional phase, the study of the timing of role losses can contribute to a better understanding of short-term as well as long-term effects of retirement and widowhood on the well-being of the elderly. In the coping or adjustment phase, the analysis of retirement attitudes, social participation, and use of health services may show that differentials in the use of these coping responses can help explain the process of aging and the need for social planning for the aged. Finally, as shown by the outcome phase, physical and social well-being in the later years can be causally determined by past and present situations.

This model is partially tested using panel data obtained from the LRHS. For example, chapter 6 presents the stability of retirement attitudes in later life and the factors that affect the continuity of these attitudes. Chapter 7 illustrates a sense of personal equilibrium in social relationships after role losses. Chapter 8 identifies the relevancy of role losses as explanatory variables for the use of physician services while other social and health factors are simultaneously considered. In addition, a targeting approach to the frail elderly is presented in this chapter, so that effective planning for health and social well-being can be made. Finally, the implications of the study findings are discussed and policy-relevant recommendations that are pertinent to health promotion and primary prevention are suggested in the last chapter.

References

1. L.K. George, *Role Transitions in Later Life* (Belmont, Calif.: Wadsworth Publishing Co., 1980).

2. T.T.H. Wan, B.G. Odell, and D.T. Lewis, *Promoting the Well-Being of the Elderly: A Community Diagnosis* (N.Y.: Haworth Press, 1982).

3. T.T.H. Wan, *Stressful Life Events, Social-Support Networks, and Gerontological Health: A Prospective Approach* (Lexington, Mass.: Lexington Books, 1982).

4. T.T.H. Wan, "Health Status, Social Support, and Use of Health Services by Functionally Disabled Elderly: LISREL Modeling Approach," in G.L. Maddox (ed.), Proceedings of the Duke University Council on Aging and Human Development Lecture Series (Durham, N.C.: Duke University, 1984).

2
Retirement Patterns

T he process of disengaging one's self from the work force through retirement is not only condoned by society but in some cases mandatory. Study of the retirement process and population is germane to social policy. Current retirement trends have increased the number of social security beneficiaries, pushing the social security system to the brink of insolvency. In addition, as the goals of public policy turn toward preserving and enhancing the quality of life of the elderly, knowledge of the process of retirement is paramount. By profiling the population as it moves from a working role into a retirement role, the key factors which characterize the retirement process can be identified and thus evaluated in terms of intervention strategies. If the adverse effects of retirement are controllable through interventions at the public policy level, then funding can be more appropriately targeted to these problems.

Related Research

Previous research on the characteristics of the retirement process and population has concluded that retirement is closely associated with age, perceived health status, and economic well-being of the retiree. What past research has failed to agree upon, however, is in exactly what way retirement is associated with age, perceived health status, and economic well-being. A number of studies have found that poor health frequently precedes and precipitates retirement [1-3]. Other studies, however, have indicated that retirement may be the agent that results in poor health [4-7]. And finally, recent research has reported contrary evidence indicating that retirement has little effect on health [3, 8, 9].

Another issue presented in many past studies on retirement is how to measure retirement. Past researchers have used objective measures to determine retirement status (level of participation in the labor force;

whether a retirement pension or social security benefits are being received) as well as a subjective measure (definitions of oneself as retired) [10, 11]. In general, the literature shows that subjective retirement status is reliably consistent with objective measures of retirement [10, 12].

Yet another area of concern where related research is minimal is the study of retirement as a process. While surveys and studies have been used to characterize retirement in terms of complete retirement, partial retirement, and nonretirement [10], longitudinal analyses profiling the retirement process, especially when concentrating on those individuals who switch from retired to nonretired, are limited.

The limitations in studying the retirement process either cross-sectionally or retrospectively are well noted [11]. Through the use of a longitudinal study sample, the present study illustrates the profiles and patterns of retirement by tracing specific age cohorts through a ten-year time span. In addition, this study identifies selected physical health and socioeconomic characteristics of the study sample as they proceed through the retirement process. From these analyses, the factors affecting retirement can be determined, and with further study policy intervention can be planned. In addition, the trend in switching from retired to nonretired is investigated. Thus, not only are we interested in why individuals retire, but we are also interested in what the stability of the retirement status is in a panel group.

Methodology

The primary data source for this analysis is the LRHS, which consists of six waves of data collected every two years from 1969 to 1979 [13]. Initially, 11,153 individuals aged fifty-eight to sixty-three responded to the 1969 survey, creating a data base containing detailed information on retirement, work history, economic status, health and functional status, as well as social and demographic attributes. Similar surveys were administered in 1971, 1973, 1975, 1977, and 1979, enabling a panel analysis to be performed which is particularly useful in studying the retirement process. The study sample (N = 6,269) for this analysis is limited to those males and nonmarried females who responded to all six surveys administered (1969–1979).

This study first analyzes the patterns of retirement by means of tracing various age cohorts (years of birth) through the years prior to and after age sixty-five. Age sixty-five is used as a benchmark as it has traditionally been the most frequent age for retirement. By analyzing retirement patterns longitudinally for specific age cohorts, a precise picture of the trend in the retirement process can be illustrated. The second part of the analysis focuses on identifying the key factors relating to retirement (a dichotomous dependent variable) through the use of logistic regression. Subjectively assessed retirement status is assigned the metric values of 0 (not retired) and 1 (retired) is the dependent variable. Age, health attributes, economic status, and prior retirement status are the independent variables.

Lastly, the stability of the retirement status is investigated. Switchers, those changing their retirement status from retired to nonretired, will also be profiled to determine those individuals who are most likely to terminate their retirement and return to work.

Results

Table 2-1 presents the percentage distributions of persons who considered themselves retired in each of the six waves of the LRHS by age cohort for males and females in 1969. About 18 percent of the male respondents and 27.5 percent of the female respondents were retired at the start of the survey in 1969. All groups of age cohorts had an increase in the number of persons considering themselves as retired. It is interesting to note that the younger birth cohorts tended to have a slightly higher proportion of retirees than the older cohorts when they reached retirement age, irrespective of gender. Moreover, a substantially larger proportion of the female respondents were retired at the preretirement age than the male respondents.

For both male and female respondents in 1969–1979, the determinants of retirement, as analyzed by logistic regression, are primarily status prior to retirement, presence of a physical disability, and age.

Table 2-2 reveals some interesting findings with regard to the relevance of selected predictors of retirement. First, retirement is positively associated with age, poor (perceived) health, and physical disability at the preretirement age (1969), irrespective of gender. Findings were similar in the later waves of the LRHS even though prior retirement status (a lagged variable) was introduced as a control variable. Second, inadequate economic resources are positively associated with retirement. However, the causal linkage between retirement and economic status cannot be ascertained in the present cross-sectional analysis. A careful assessment of the cause-effect relationship between these two variables needs to be undertaken so that the consequence of retirement for economic well-being can be determined. Third, education level is negatively associated with retirement: the higher the education level one has attained, the less likely one will retire at or after retirement age. This

Table 2-1
Percentage Distributions of Persons Who Retired before Age 65 and at Retirement Age in Six Waves of the Retirement History Study by Age Cohort in 1969

Age in 1969 (birth cohort)	1969	1971	1973	1975	1977	1979
Male Panel[a]						
58 (1911)	8.9	15.8	39.1	58.8	85.8	89.6
59 (1910)	11.2	18.9	43.1	76.1	87.7	91.2
60 (1909)	15.1	32.8	56.0	84.4	90.8	93.8
61 (1908)	19.4	41.8	75.4	87.0	90.5	93.3
62 (1907)	25.4	47.2	79.7	88.5	93.5	95.3
63 (1906)	32.6	68.1	82.9	89.8	92.0	93.0
Total (1906–1911)	17.8	35.8	71.6	79.9	89.9	92.6
Female Panel[b]						
58 (1911)	17.4	36.6	58.6	69.7	86.8	89.5
59 (1910)	18.0	38.8	56.1	77.9	85.1	90.7
60 (1909)	23.2	50.2	66.6	87.8	93.6	95.8
61 (1908)	31.2	58.2	78.1	86.5	89.7	90.7
62 (1907)	36.5	63.5	78.3	88.3	92.2	93.1
63 (1906)	44.5	74.7	86.4	91.9	92.2	95.8
Total (1906–1911)	27.5	54.1	70.5	83.7	89.9	92.5

Note: The figure underlined represents the percentage of persons who retired at or after the retirement age (65).
[a]N = 4,385.
[b]N = 1,884.

relationship is particularly marked among male respondents. Fourth, status prior to retirement bears a strong positive effect on the later retirement status. This suggests that relative stability of retirement status is observed among older adults; those who are retired are likely to remain retired in later life. These findings are consistent with previously cited related research.

Switchers of Retirement Status

Although retirement is considered a relatively static phenomenon among the elderly, some retirees do return to work in later life for a variety of reasons. Little is known about the magnitude and nature of this switching behavior, however. The questions which need to be answered are: First, are there any significant differences in social and health char-

Table 2–2
Logistic Regression of the Conditional Probability of Retirement on Selected Predictors and Prior Retirement Status (Lagged Variable)

	1969		1971		1973		1975		1977	
	Male	Female	Male	Female	Male	Female	Male	Female	Male	Female
	Probability of Retirement (Beta Coefficient)									
Predictors										
Education	-0.01	-0.08	-0.11[a]	-0.25[a]	-0.21[a]	-0.04	-0.26[a]	0.13	-0.23[a]	0.17
Age	0.36[a]	0.34[a]	0.49[a]	0.31[a]	0.35[a]	0.17[a]	0.16[a]	0.18[a]	-0.14[a]	-0.07
NPH	1.02[a]	0.49[a]	0.12	0.13	-0.10	0.41[a]	0.10	0.25	0.13	0.40
DIS	1.51[a]	1.00[a]	1.18[a]	1.09[a]	1.07[a]	0.49[a]	0.58[a]	0.36[a]	0.82[a]	0.76[a]
ECON	0.53[a]	0.31[a]	0.51[a]	0.65[a]	0.33	0.52[a]	0.47[a]	0.67[a]	-0.04	0.13
UNHAP	0.33[a]	0.26	0.30[a]	-0.14	0.25	-0.06	-0.05	0.07	0.28	-0.14
RET	—	—	3.25[a]	2.34	2.56[a]	2.70[a]	3.40[a]	2.60[a]	3.50[a]	2.95[a]
N	4,124	1,717	4,241	1,813	3,809	1,822	4,323	1,860	4,295	1,844
Overall model fit (χ^2)	885	256	1,945	652	929	650	1,531	447	1,004	335
R^2 (%)	22.66	19.54	34.92	25.50	27.35	34.93	26.21	35.28	35.28	26.63

Note: NPH–presence (1) or absence (0) of deterioration in self-assessed health.
DIS–presence (1) or absence (0) of a physical disability.
ECON–inadequate (1) or adequate (0) economic resources.
UNHAP–unhappiness (1) or happiness (0) of life.
RET–retired (1) or nonretired (1) in the prior survey period.

[a]$p < .05$.

acteristics between switchers (those switched from retired to nonretired status) and nonswitchers? Second, can we predict the switching behavior?

Based upon LRHS data, only 658 of 6,269 respondents studied switched retirement status even once in the ten-year period. Approximately 2–3 percent of respondents were switchers for each of the five waves (1971–1979). Data in table 2–3 show that no significant age difference between switchers and nonswitchers was observed. A substantially higher proportion of male respondents was found among nonswitchers than among switchers. Overall, the switched tended to perceive their economic status to be worse than the nonswitched. Before 1977, no statistically significant differences were found between switchers and nonswitchers. However, during and after this period the switchers tended to perceive themselves as having better health than the nonswitchers.

Findings thus far in this analysis have indicated that individuals are more likely to switch from a retired status to a nonretired status if they are females and if they perceive their economic status as inadequate in earlier retirement years. A hypothesis can be postulated that the initial retirement decision is not a terminal event, rather a process whereby some individuals may move back and forth from a retired to nonretired status. The reasons for this pattern can be better identified by employing logistic regression analysis of switching behavior in terms of their health and socioeconomic characteristics.

Through the use of logistic regression analysis, the determinants of a switch from retired to not retired are shown in table 2–4. The key determinants are age, sex, economic well-being, and health status. Female respondents were more likely to switch than male respondents. Disability (the disabled coded 1 and others coded 0) is negatively related to switching retirement status, while poor economic well-being is positively related to switching status. This makes intuitive sense, as the lower one's economic well-being sinks, the more reason one has to return to work. We found that even as age advances, diminished economic well-being increases the chance that an elder will switch from retired to nonretired status if health permits.

Further analysis of the retirement switching phenomenon for the male and female samples revealed that the findings remain consistent with the total sample, as economic well-being and physical health continue to be the most influential factors contributing to switches from retired to nonretired status. Of interest here is that persons free of physical disability are more likely to switch from retired to nonretired status. Economic resources, however, seem less important than physical disability in predicting a switch from retired to nonretired status.

Table 2-3
Mean Distributions of Selected Social and Health Characteristics of a Panel of Older Adults by Switched Retirement Status (Retired to Nonretired) by Survey Year
(N = 6,269)

Year/Switched Status	Mean Age	Percent Male	Percent Unhappy	Percent Poor Economic Well-Being	Percent Poor Health	Percent Disabled
1971–1979						
Switched (N = 5,605)	—	58.8[a]	17.6	20.0[a]	23.7	33.9
Nonswitched (N = 658)	—	71.3[a]	15.2	14.2[a]	26.0	32.6
1971						
Switched (N = 6,057)	62.4	55.4[a]	13.0	20.0	25.0	39.1
Nonswitched (N = 115)	62.5	70.3[a]	15.5	14.7	25.7	32.6
1973						
Switched (N = 6,122)	64.8	56.4[a]	22.4	23.2[a]	26.1	41.4
Nonswitched (N = 131)	64.4	70.4[a]	17.1	13.8[a]	28.9	38.4
1975						
Switched (N = 6,138)	66.3	50.4[a]	22.4	13.6	28.6	32.3
Nonswitched (N = 131)	66.5	70.4[a]	17.1	13.4	28.1	37.4
1977						
Switched (N = 6,130)	68.6	58.3[a]	17.3	18.0	25.0[a]	32.8[a]
Nonswitched (N = 139)	68.4	70.2[a]	18.1	14.7	31.6[a]	43.8[a]
1979						
Switched (N = 6,077)	70.1	67.7[a]	13.8	12.7	26.3[a]	26.7[a]
Nonswitched (N = 157)	70.4	70.0[a]	18.7	15.0	34.4[a]	49.5[a]

[a]Significant at 0.05 or lower level for the mean difference between the switched and nonswitched retirement status.

Table 2–4
Logistic Regression of the Conditional Probability of Switching from Retired to Nonretired Status on Selected Predictors

Predictors	1971 Beta	1971 R	1973 Beta	1973 R	1975 Beta	1975 R	1977 Beta	1977 R	1979 Beta	1979 R
Education	-0.18	-0.01	-0.37ᵃ	-0.08	-0.12	0.00	-0.20	-0.03	-0.12	0.00
Age	0.00	0.00	0.13ᵃ	0.05	-0.06	0.00	0.08	0.01	-0.10ᵃ	-0.04
Sex	-0.67ᵃ	-0.10	-0.58ᵃ	-0.08	0.90ᵃ	-0.14	-0.61ᵃ	-0.09	-0.16	0.00
NPH	-0.23	0.00	-0.32	0.00	-0.00	0.00	-0.30	0.00	0.02	0.00
DIS	0.35	0.03	-0.06	0.00	-0.22	0.00	-0.47ᵃ	-0.05	-1.01ᵃ	-0.13
ECON	0.22	0.00	0.48ᵃ	0.05	-0.14	0.00	0.30	0.00	0.05	0.00
UNHAP	-0.38	0.00	0.24	0.00	-0.02	0.00	0.01	0.00	-0.09	0.00
N	6,054		4,631		6,183		6,139		6,129	
Fit (χ^2)	20.0		29.2		26.1		26.2		39.8	
R^2 (%)	0.53		1.37		1.00		0.98		1.80	

Note: Sex–male coded 1 and female coded 0.
NPH–presence (1) or absence (0) of deterioration in health.
DIS–presence (1) or absence (0) of a physical disability.
ECON–inadequate (1) or adequate (0) economic resources.
UNHAP–unhappiness (1) or happiness (0).
Switching status–switcher (1) or nonswitcher (0) of retirement status.
ᵃ$p < .05$.

Conclusions

In conclusion, in our analysis of those individuals that initially retired and then resumed employment in the early retirement years (age sixty-five and under), we found that gender was the most important attribute. Findings seem to indicate that as persons reach the traditional retirement age of sixty-five they may retire because they have always planned and wanted to retire, but that some needed to return to work due to economic considerations in the earlier periods (before 1975). Thus, the movement from retired to nonretired status further provides evidence that for some individuals retirement is very much a process and not a nonreversible event.

The implications of these analyses are that older individuals, approaching retirement and also in need of economic resources, are likely to be able to remain in the work force and help provide for themselves. This finding may suggest policy decisions on both the timing and level of social security benefits. For example, moving the age at which benefits are realized may be one option; instituting a system of graduated benefits may be another. Furthermore, any intervention strategies that promote the well-being of the elderly during the earlier periods of their aging process will greatly facilitate their decision to resume employment if they feel they need it.

References

1. R.C. Atchley and J.L. Robinson, "Attitudes Toward Retirement and Distance from the Event," *Research on Aging* 4 (1982):299–313.

2. L.K. George and G.L. Maddox, "Subjective Adaptation to Loss of the Work Role: A Longitudinal Study," *Journal of Gerontology* 32 (1977):456–462.

3. E.B. Palmore, G.G. Fillenbaum, and L.K. George, "Consequences of Retirement," *Journal of Gerontology* 39 (1984):109–116.

4. W. Casscells, D. Evans, R.A. DeSilva, J.E. Davies, C.H. Hennekens, B. Rosener, B. Lown, and M.J. Jesse, "Retirement and Coronary Mortality," *The Lancet* 1, no. 8181 (1980):1288–1289.

5. D.J. Ekerdt and R. Bosse, "Change in Self-Reported Health with Retirement," *International Journal of Aging and Human Development* 15 (1982): 213–223.

6. E.R. Gonzalez, "Retiring May Predispose to Fatal Heart Attack," *Journal of American Medical Association* 243 (1980):13–14.

7. J. Martin and A. Doran, "Evidence Concerning the Relationship Between Health and Retirement," *Sociological Review* 14 (1966):329–343.

8. D.J. Ekerdt, L. Baden, R. Bosse, and E. Dibbs, "The Effect of Retirement on Physical Health," *American Journal of Public Health* 73 (1983): 779–783.

9. L.K. George, G.G. Fillenbaum, and E.B. Palmore, "Sex Differences in the Antecedents and Consequences of Retirement," *Journal of Gerontology* 39 (1984):364–371.

10. J. Murray, "Subjective Retirement," *Social Security Bulletin* 42 (1979): 20–25.

11. E.B. Palmore, L.K. George, and G.G. Fillenbaum, "Predictors of Retirement," *Journal of Gerontology* 37 (1982):733–742.

12. A. Foner and K. Schwab, *Aging and Retirement* (Monterey, Calif.: Brooks/Cole Publishing Co., 1980).

13. L.M. Irelan and K. Schwab, "The Social Security Administration Retirement History Study," *Research on Aging* 3 (1981):381–386.

3
Widowhood

The increased longevity that has resulted from improved social and environmental circumstances is not without consequence, for as medical and technological advances extend the life span, the likelihood of widowhood increases. Although widowhood can occur at any time during adulthood, this event is more devastating to the elderly. Faced with reduced income, deteriorating health, and a dwindling social network, the elderly are frequently less prepared to deal with it. The impact of widowhood must be identified in order to design strategies that can counteract the adverse effects of this stressful event.

Related Research

Previous studies have found that widowhood negatively affects physical, psychological, and social well-being. Of five role losses studied, Wan [1] identified widowhood as the most important predictor of poor health. Widowhood and retirement, occurring concomitantly, were also found to be disabling. The mourning process which follows the loss of a spouse can lead to serious bodily dysfunctions [2, 3]. Increased morbidity and higher mortality have been observed for the widowed during the year following the loss of the spouse [3-5].

Psychological complaints increased after this loss, with the widowed exhibiting lower morale [6, 7] and more symptoms associated with depression [8] than married persons. The observed level of life satisfaction for the recently widowed decreased to levels associated with experiencing three or more health problems [9]. A significant change in attitudes toward work and usefulness was reported for male and female widowed, respectively [10]. In addition, males were found to suffer from identity problems due to the loss of their role as husband [11].

Several studies found that widowhood affects psychological well-being to a greater degree than physical health [8, 12, 13]. Changes that were noted may be due, however, not to the role loss itself but to adjustments to new roles that must be assumed [14]. The health status concern of the widowed may be due to concomitant changes in financial, environmental, and social factors, in addition to the loss of spouse [13, 15, 16].

Widowhood has a negative impact on income, especially for females. Following widowhood, real family income decreases substantially. Income inadequacy has been found to have a direct and negative effect on health [15], transportation [11], and social interaction [15, 17]. In addition, the income of the widowed has a positive relationship with life satisfaction [9]. The impact of income on these economic, social, and health factors should be considered in determining the full effect of widowhood on the elderly.

It is well recognized that the widowed should not be considered as a homogeneous group. Differences in the impact of widowhood exist between widower and widow, as was stated above. Females are thought to be at greater economic risk while males experience greater health deterioration following widowhood. While widows experience increased family interaction [16], Lopata [15] details several factors which give widowers social advantages over widows.

Besides income and gender, other factors must be considered when studying the widowed elderly. Age has been found to affect psychological well-being [4] and perceived health status [18]. Heyman and Gianturco [10] found that age could explain reported declines in health and life style associated with widowhood. Multiple role losses such as widowhood and retirement have been found to occur with advanced age. Experiencing these multiple events can produce cumulative effects [19, 20], frequently placing additional strain on existing resources. Additionally, widowhood has been found to affect social participation, both directly and indirectly, through variables such as health, income, and education [21, 22].

Methodology

A descriptive analysis was performed based on data obtained from the LRHS for the years 1969, 1971, 1973, 1975, 1977, and 1979 to observe characteristics of the widowed elderly. During each of these six years a survey was administered to the initial 1969 sample (N = 11,153) to gather information on physical health, socioeconomic background, work experience, morale, and marital status of older adult males and nonmarried females. Those members of the 1969 sample who responded to all of the surveys constitute the sample (N = 6,269) for this analysis.

It consists of 4,385 males and 1,884 females aged fifty-eight to sixty-three in 1969.

A one-way analysis of variance was employed to examine the effect of widowhood (the widowed coded 1 and non-widowed 0) on each of the three indicators of well-being (happiness, health deterioration, and adequacy of economic resources).

Results

Widowhood by Gender

Table 3–1 shows the number of persons who reported being widowed in each wave of the study. As expected, the number of widowed increased as the population aged, so that by 1979, when the respondents were between sixty-eight and seventy-three years old, 26.2 percent of the sample population were widowed. It should be noted that this figure is higher than the national figure for widowed persons in this age category [23].

More females than males experienced widowhood since unmarried females (including widows) were selected in the beginning of the survey. By the last wave, 66 percent of the female respondents were widowed as compared to 9.2 percent of their male counterparts. Although females are expected to outnumber males within age ranks of the widowed, our finding may be due to the predominance of males in the original sample.

Although not specifically indicated on any table, an analysis was completed to determine whether the respondents tended to remarry. Because of the age of the sample, it was expected that the probability of remarriage would be low, approximately 5 percent for females and 25 percent for males [24]. Our analysis for LRHS data from 1975 through 1979 found that only a very small proportion of the study population remarried. This finding held regardless of gender.

Health Effects of Widowhood

The impact of widowhood on physical health was examined. The widowed were asked whether their physical health was better or worse compared with that of two years ago. A slightly larger percentage of widowers reported a lower level of physical well-being, although the effect of widowhood on them was not statistically significant (table 3–2). More of the widows reported a decline in health than nonwidows in all six waves of the study. It is interesting to note that the proportion of

Table 3–1
Proportion and Number of Persons by Widowhood Status in the Survey Years, 1969–1979

Survey Year	Total (N = 6,269)				Male (N = 4,385)				Female (N = 1,884)			
	Widowed		Nonwidowed		Widowed		Nonwidowed		Widowed		Nonwidowed	
	N	%	N	%	N	%	N	%	N	%	N	%
1969	1,389	22.2	4,880	77.8	152	3.5	4,233	96.5	1,237	65.7	647	34.2
1971	1,418	22.6	4,851	77.4	198	4.5	4,187	95.5	1,220	64.8	664	35.2
1973	1,450	23.1	4,819	76.9	229	5.2	4,156	94.8	1,221	64.8	663	35.2
1975	1,502	24.0	4,767	76.0	272	6.2	4,113	93.8	1,230	65.3	654	34.7
1977	1,580	25.2	4,689	74.8	335	7.6	4,050	92.4	1,245	66.1	639	33.9
1979	1,644	26.2	4,625	73.8	404	9.2	3,981	90.8	1,240	65.8	644	34.2

Table 3–2
Mean (Percentage) Distributions of Selected Well-Being Indicators of Older Males by Widowhood Status and Its Effect

| | Effect on the Well-Being Indicators | | | | | |
| | Health Deterioration | | Poor Economically | | Unhappy Life | |
Year/Widowhood Status	%	N	%	N	%	N
1969						
Widowed	25.2	148	13.2	151	17.3	150
Nonwidowed	21.6	4,136	11.4	4,165	13.5	4,177
			Effect on 1971 Measures			
1971						
Widowed	28.2	195	12.8	4,129	16.6	2,721
Nonwidowed	24.6	4,085	11.4	4,129	16.6	2,721
			Effect on 1973 Measures			
1973						
Widowed	26.9	228	14.0	229	25.9[a]	228
Nonwidowed	25.9	4,148	11.2	4,133	17.0[a]	4,139
			Effect on 1975 Measures			
1975						
Widowed	28.5	270	17.8[a]	270	23.1[a]	268
Nonwidowed	30.0	4,093	12.5[a]	4,088	17.3[a]	4,056
			Effect on 1977 Measures			
1977						
Widowed	34.1	334	17.6[a]	335	22.8[a]	328
Nonwidowed	33.2	4,040	13.1[a]	4,030	18.4[a]	3,982
			Effect on 1979 Measures			

Note: N = Total number of individuals studied.
[a]Significant at 0.05 or lower level for the mean difference between widowed and nonwidowed persons.

health deterioration increased as the panel aged, irrespective of gender (table 3-3). This is the result of the natural aging process which is frequently accompanied by deteriorating health and increased disability.

The widowed demonstrated a consistently higher percentage of health deterioration than the nonwidowed. This is true for both sexes in all waves of the study. However, sex differentials exist in the levels of reported physical well-being, with widowhood having a greater impact on females than males.

These findings do not imply that widowhood causes poor health since prior health of the widowed is not considered in this analysis. However, detailed multivariate analysis of widowhood effects will be examined in later chapters.

Widowhood and Socioeconomic Well-Being

Socioeconomic well-being is determined by two indicators: (1) the adequacy of economic resources perceived by the elderly, and (2) the presence or absence of happiness of life. Both widow and widower exhibited significant differences in social and economic well-being. The widowed had a higher proportion of persons reporting poor economic status and unhappiness (tables 3-2 and 3-3). These differences became much more pronounced after 1973. For males, widowhood appeared to have more adverse effects on their social and economic well-being in the later periods (1977 and 1979), while for females the widowhood effect tended to appear in the earlier periods.

Widowhood had a negative impact on average family income for both male and female widowed when we examined the total family income of the study population. However, widows are at a greater disadvantage than widowers since the former consistently had lower average family incomes than the latter. This is not surprising because the husband is usually the breadwinner, and the loss of his earnings would be expected to have greater impact on family income.

Widowhood was found to have a negative impact on perceived happiness. Considering the effect of widowhood on physical health and economic status, this result was not unexpected. The decreased levels of physical well-being of the widowed are also reflected in these findings. Widows, in all waves where data were available, were more likely to report having inadequate economic resources than widowers. In later periods of the study, we found that more widowers tended to perceive having an unhappy life than widows.

Table 3–3
Mean (Percentage) Distributions of Selected Well-Being Indicators of Older Females by Widowhood Status and Its Effect

| | *Effect on the Well-Being Indicators* | | | | | |
| | *Health Deterioration* | | *Poor Economically* | | *Unhappy Life* | |
Year/Widowhood Status	%	N	%	N	%	N
			Effect on 1971 Measures			
1969						
Widowed	28.7[a]	1,207	22.6	1,219	18.9	1,224
Nonwidowed	24.2[a]	625	22.6	637	21.0	642
			Effect on 1973 Measures			
1971						
Widowed	32.8[a]	1,200	20.6	1,204	18.8	1,215
Nonwidowed	26.5[a]	653	18.3	654	16.8	661
			Effect on 1975 Measures			
1973						
Widowed	32.8[a]	1,218	19.7[a]	1,216	20.9[a]	1,216
Nonwidowed	28.2[a]	660	15.3[a]	659	15.7[a]	657
			Effect on 1977 Measures			
1975						
Widowed	36.1	1,225	21.2[a]	1,224	19.5	1,211
Nonwidowed	33.2	651	15.4[a]	649	18.6	646
			Effect on 1979 Measures			
1977						
Widowed	38.0[a]	1,239	19.4	1,238	19.5[a]	1,229
Nonwidowed	33.0[a]	636	16.3	631	15.0[a]	634

Note: N = Total number of individuals studied.
[a]Significant at 0.05 or lower level for the mean difference between widowed and nonwidowed persons.

Conclusions

The study findings appear to confirm that widowhood has an adverse effect on the elderly. While its impact is felt by both widow and widower, more widows experience a decline in health due to widowhood than do widowers. Widows, also, are at an increased risk of economic deprivation, as they have the lowest income level of all groups studied. Unhappiness is also a result of widowhood and is experienced to a greater degree by widowers in the later periods of the study.

Although the repeated cross-sectional analysis of the relationship of widowhood to health and socioeconomic conditions of older adults indicates a possible adverse effect of widowhood on these conditions, this finding needs to be substantiated by performing multivariate analysis, controlling for the effect of prior health and socioeconomic conditions. Thus, a panel analysis of the study sample is called for. Otherwise, the relationship between widowhood of the elderly and these conditions can not be fully determined. Detailed causal analysis of the structural relationship between widowhood and well-being of the elderly is presented in chapters 4 and 5.

References

1. T.H. Wan, *Stressful Life Events, Social-Support Networks and Gerontological Health: A Prospective Approach* (Lexington, Mass.: Lexington Books, 1982).

2. G.H. Pollack, "Mourning and Adaptation," *International Journal of Psychoanalysis* 42 (1961):341–361.

3. M. Young, B. Benjamin, and C. Wallis, "The Mortality of Widowers," *The Lancet* 2 (1963):454–456.

4. C. Parkes, B. Benjamin, and R.G. Fitzgerald, "Broken Heart: A Statistical Study of Increased Mortality Among Widowers," *British Medical Journal* 1 (1969):740–743.

5. K.F. Rowland, "Environmental Events Predicting Death for the Elderly," *Psychological Bulletin* 84 (1977):349–372.

6. L.K. George, *Role Transitions in Later Life* (Monterey, Calif.: Brooks/Cole Publishing Co., 1980).

7. L.A. Morgan, "Changes in Family Interaction Following Widowhood," *Journal of Marriage and Family* 46 (1983):323–332.

8. P.J. Clayton, "Mortality and Morbidity in the First Year of Widowhood," *Archives of General Psychiatry* 30 (1974):747–750.

9. H. Beck, "Adjustment to and Satisfaction with Retirement," *Journal of Gerontology* 37 (1982):616–624.

10. D.K. Heyman and D.T. Gianturco, "Long-Term Adaptation by the Elderly to Bereavement," *Journal of Gerontology* 28 (1973):359–362.

11. R.C. Atchley, "Dimensions of Widowhood in Later Life," *The Gerontologist* 15 (1975):175–178.

12. D. Maddison and A. Viola, "The Health of Widows in the Year Following Bereavement," *Journal of Psychosomatic Research* 12 (1968):297–306.

13. C.M. Parkes, "Effects of Bereavement on Physical and Mental Health— A Study of the Medical Records of Widows," *British Journal of Medicine* 2 (1964):274–279.

14. L.I. Pearlin and M.A. Lieberman, "Social Sources of Emotional Distress," *Research in Community and Mental Health* 1 (1979):217–248.

15. H.Z. Lopata, "Widows as a Minority Group," *The Gerontologist* 11 (1971):67–77.

16. L.A. Morgan, "A Re-examination of Widowhood and Morale," *Journal of Gerontology* 31 (1976):687–695.

17. K.F. Ferraro, E. Mutran, and C.M. Barresi, "Widowhood, Health, and Friendship Support in Later Life," *Journal of Health and Social Behavior* 25 (1984):246–259.

18. W.C. Cockerham, K. Sharp, and J. Wilcox, "Aging and Perceived Health Status," *Journal of Gerontology* 38 (1983):349–355.

19. E.B. Palmore, W.P. Cleveland, J.B. Nowlin, D.F. Ramm, and I. Siegler, "Stress and Adaptation in Later Life," *Journal of Gerontology* 34 (1979): 841–851.

20. D.E. Stull and L.R. Hatch, "Unravelling the Effects of Multiple Life Changes," *Research on Aging* 6 (1984):560–571.

21. T.T.H. Wan and B.G. Odell, "Major Role Losses and Social Participation of Older Males," *Research on Aging* 5 (1983):173–196.

22. K.F. Ferraro, "Widowhood and Social Participation in Later Life: Isolation or Compensation?," *Research on Aging* 6 (1984):451–468.

23. U.S. Bureau of the Census, *Marital Status and Living Arrangements: March 1982*, Current Population Reports, Series P-20, No. 38 (Washington, D.C.: U.S. Government Printing Office, 1983).

24. W.P. Cleveland and D.T. Gianturco, "Remarriage Probability After Widowhood: A Retrospective Method," *Journal of Gerontology* 31 (1976): 99–103.

4

Health Consequences of Major Role
Losses in Later Life

T he loss of work and family-related roles may occur concomitantly in the last stage of life [1–3]. These life-change events may be conceptualized as stressful events which have deleterious effects on the well-being of individuals, including decline in life satisfaction, deterioration of perceived health and physical functioning, and an increase in morbidity and mortality risk. Although gerontological researchers have reported little health effects due to retirement [4, 5], others have noted that the coincidence of multiple role losses, such as retirement and widowhood occurring within a given period, may have a negative influence on an individual's well-being in later life [1, 6, 7].

Most previous research on life events has concentrated on cross-sectional surveys of psychological and physiological attributes of young adults [8–10]. Little has been done using a longitudinal approach to assess the differential impact of the timing of life events on the physical well-being of a panel of older adults. There have been a few longitudinal studies of the health consequences of retirement and widowhood, but most of these studies use a retrospective rather than a prospective approach [11, 12]. Thus, the causal relationship between life events and gerontological health cannot be fully ascertained. Furthermore, the long-term cumulative impact of major life events on physical and mental well-being needs to be demonstrated so that scientific preventive strategies can be developed for the most likely to be adversely affected by changes in work status, marital status, and other family-related roles.

This research is to examine the effect of cumulative losses experienced by older adults in later life. Loss of work role through involuntary retirement and loss of spouse may adversely affect health and well-

A reprint from T.T.H. Wan, "Health Consequences of Major Role Losses in Later Life," *Research on Aging* 6 (1984):469–489. Reprinted by permission of Sage Publications, Inc.

being of the elderly if no adequate coping resources or supportive mechanisms are available. In order to adequately understand and prepare for successful aging, it is imperative to systematically examine the causal sequence of role loss and its health effects, while social and demographic characteristics of the elderly are simultaneously taken into account.

This chapter will address several key issues pertaining to the causal relationship between health and concomitant role losses. First, what are the health consequences of major role losses? Second, what are health and social characteristics of those who are likely to experience multiple role losses? Third, what are specific coping responses of the elderly who have experienced multiple role losses? Finally, what are the mechanisms for reducing the risk of being adversely affected by the experience of concomitant role losses such as retirement and widowhood?

Related Research

The Health Consequences of Retirement

Generally, retirement is defined as the point at which an individual decides to withdraw from the active work role and has no intent to seek other employment. Some older adults retire due to illness or disability while others are involuntarily removed from the work force for non-health reasons. Despite the fact that persons may retire for different, and in some cases multiple, reasons, the effect of either voluntary or involuntary retirement on an individual's health deserves systematic research.

Previous research has documented that some persons enjoyed improved health after retirement, indicating a positive outcome of retirement [3]. In comparing retired and working men, Martin and Doran [14] reported that men over age fifty-five showed steadily increasing incidences of serious illness with advancing age, but those who had compulsory retirement at the retirement age experienced lower incidences of serious illness.

The retirement process, which is so often the portal through which the adaptation to role loss starts, can easily become the precipitating agent for physical and psychological disorders. This theoretical assumption has dominated previous empirical studies, focusing on stressful life events and their adverse effects [15]. The interpretation of the pathogenesis of recent life events can be found in much of the literature of psychosomatic medicine [1]. According to Cassel [16], social factors such as role loss may increase the risk of ill health by increasing the general susceptibility to disease. In an investigation of the relationship between normal involuntary retirement and early mortality among rubber workers, Haynes and her associates [17] reported that increased mortality risk was observed in the first three years of retirement among those who were forced to retire, particularly among persons with low social status. Clinical evidence has been found by Casscells and his associates [18] which indicates that the risk of coronary heart disease mortality may be directly linked to retirement. They reported that those who retired had a substantially higher mortality risk than those who did not retire. Similarly, in a case-control study of 1,136 males, Gonzalez [19] also found that fatal heart attacks were more prevalent among the retired than the nonretired. Two recent studies on health services utilization of the adult population showed that the retired had a higher utilization rate of physician services and spent more for medical care than the nonretired [20, 21].

The above studies pointed out the potential harmful effect of retirement and its consequences due to maladaption. These studies, however, were plagued by a common methodological flaw because they lacked proper statistical control of selectivity factors and their analyses were limited by a retrospective study design.

In order to improve the understanding of the effects of retirement on health status, recent studies have taken a prospective approach to avoid selectivity bias and to control for extraneous factors that may confound the true relationship between health and retirement [1, 22]. Based upon panel data obtained from the first four of six waves of the LRHS, Wan [1] employed a prospective study design to compare pre- to postretirement changes in the physical health of older adults who were working and had no physical incapacities or disabling conditions in the initial study period. Controlling for the prior health status of the panel, Wan found that retirement per se did not significantly affect self-assessed health status and functional capacities, but the concomitance of stressful life events—such as retirement, widowhood, and other role changes—were associated with the deterioration of health. In the analysis of data from the Veterans Administration Normative Aging Study, Ekerdt and his associates [22] reported that retirement did not influence the risk of health deterioration, nor did it exert any positive effect on physical health as measured by both self-assessed and clinically assessed indicators of health. These findings, derived from longitudinal studies, have been further substantiated by Palmore and his associates [6] in their comparative analysis of panel data from three national (the National Longitudinal Survey, the LRHS, and the Panel Study of Income Dynamics) and three local (the Duke Second Longitudinal Study, the Duke Work and Retirement Study, and the Ohio Longitudinal Study) studies.

The Health Consequences of Widowhood

The loss of spouse role through widowhood may disrupt the life pattern of the suvivors and result in an immediate decrease in their perceived health status [23]. The acute stage of mourning has several phases including shock, grief, pain, and the initial steps of "letting go" and is followed by the chronic stage where readaptation to life occurs [24]. Mourning involves depression or melancholia, but the shock can be so serious as to cause somatic dysfunction. Previous empirical findings have consistently indicated that the health of the widowed or widowers is adversely affected by the experience of widowhood [25–27].

Maddison and Viola [26] discovered that there were more complaints about health in widows between the ages of forty-five and fifty-nine years than among a comparable nonbereaved group. Heyman and Giantarco [28], however, have refuted such claims and found that widowed persons experience only time-related health deterioration. Likewise, Elwell and Maltbie-Crannell [29] concluded that the effect of widowhood on self-assessed health was indirect, mediated through income status.

Young and his associates [30], in a study of the effect of duration of widowhood on mortality, reported that excess mortality rates in the first six months of widowhood were observed, with widowers having a 40 percent greater chance of death than married men. However, after the first six months mortality rates dropped back to normal. In comparing pre- to postwidowhood changes in health, Parkes [31] indicated that both psychiatric and nonpsychiatric complaints increased after bereavement. Furthermore, six months after bereavement, the rate of psychiatric complaints returned to the prebereavement level while the rate of nonpsychiatric complaints remained elevated, particularly among the elderly.

In a case-control study of mortality and morbidity in the first year of widowhood, Clayton [32] found that the widowed experienced more symptoms associated with depression, shortness of breath, and palpitation than members of the control group (the married). Similarly, Clayton and her associates [33] revealed that widows and widowers shared certain common symptoms of bereavement, but widows experience more sleep disturbance than widowers.

Evidence to date reveals that the widowed have a higher rate of somatic illnesses, psychiatric symptoms, and mortality than the married. However, contrary to most of the studies cited, the single positive finding was a report of elders who adapted well to bereavement, with little health change occurring after widowhood [28]. The authors justified this finding by stating that their study sample was relatively homogenous with respect to age (most of the subjects were seventy years or older).

The Synergistic Effect of Retirement and Widowhood

The effect of major role losses on health may be cumulative, since loss of two or more roles simultaneously may generate added deteriorative effects. Research has shown that the clustering of the multiple life-change events may be considered as a necessary but not sufficient cause of illness and may account in part for the time of onset of disease [34–37].

In the analyses of the Duke Longitudinal Study data, Palmore and his associates [5] reported that multiple events including retirement, widowhood, spouse's retirement, major medical problems, and departure of last child from home tended to exert cumulative effects on the well-being of the elderly. This finding was confirmed by several recent empirical studies [1, 38–39].

Methodology

Data Source

Disaggregate (individual) data obtained from the LRHS of 11,153 older adults since 1969 are the primary source for this research. The panel analysis used data from the years 1969, 1971, 1973, 1975, 1977 and 1979 of the LRHS. Detailed information pertaining to retirement, work history, economic status, pension benefits, health and functional status, and many social demographic attributes are available for panel analysis.

Sample Design

The original sample of the 1969 LRHS consisted of 11,153 persons, aged fifty-eight to sixty-three, who were either (1) married and unmarried men or (2) nonmarried women. These individuals constituted a sample drawn by stratified random cluster sampling procedures as used in the current population survey of the Bureau of the Census. The 1971 LRHS follow-up survey interviewed 9,924 persons previously surveyed in 1969, plus 245 surviving spouses. By 1973, the second follow-up survey reinterviewed 8,928 individuals. Of the 2,225 persons who were not interviewed, 984 were deaths and the remainder either refused to participate or could not be located. There were 8,716 interviewed in 1975; of these, 727 were with surviving spouses of original respondents who died sometime after 1969. In 1977, there were 7,079 interviews completed from the original study sample. In 1979, 6,270 original sampled individuals and 1,082 surviving spouses were reinterviewed.

Housewives of the cohort, whose retirement is often linked to that of their husbands, were intentionally excluded as primary respondents.

Information was obtained on the work experience, attitudes, and morale of the wives of married men in the sample. If the male respondent died, their widows were continued in the study.

From the initial sample, those who had completed information about their physical health, socioeconomic background, retirement history, and marital status throughout the ten-year study period were selected. Furthermore, the study sample was restricted to those who had worked before 1969 and remained alive in 1977. A total number of 2,476 persons is the basis of the present analysis, including 1,804 males and 672 females. Since the focus of this study is on the health impacts of major role losses in later life, the male and female samples, which varied in health status and in other characteristics during the initial study period, were analyzed separately.

Measurement

Two endogenous (latent) variables were used: physical health in 1977 and physical health in 1979. Physical health was operationally defined in terms of perceived health (poor health coded 1 and others coded 0), chronic disorder (presence of a function-limiting condition coded 1 and absence of disorder coded 0), and limitations in mobility (incapacity coded 1 and no incapacity coded 0).

Five exogenous variables used in the analysis included: age (X_1), recency of retirement (X_2), recency of widowhood (X_3), total annual income (X_4), and total number of physician contacts in 1975. Retirement was a self-reported status and further validated by responses to questions about labor force participation. Those who reported themselves as retired but still participated in the work force were treated as not retired. Since retirement at a given time was considered as a discrete variable for each wave of the LRHS, a pattern of retirement emerged from the combination of retirement status for multiple waves. For instance, during the five waves (eight years) of the LRHS study, an individual might have maintained the same retirement status, either never retired (scored 0) or completely retired throughout five waves (scored 4). The individual who retired in the fifth wave (1977) of the study was assigned a score of 1 (the most recently or newly retired). Those who retired in the third or fourth wave and remained retired throughout the rest of the study were assigned a score of 3 and 2, respectively. This variable allowed us to measure the timing and duration of retirement of the study sample.

Widowhood as a major role loss can be identified from the reported marital status in the study periods. The timing and duration of widowhood can be coded as follows:

Widowhood Status in Five Waves	Code
Never widowed	0
Recently widowed (1977)	1
Widowed since 1975	2
Widowed since 1973	3
Widowed since 1971	4

The income variable, a social class indicator, was measured by the annual income of 1975. However, its distribution was very skewed so that a log transformation was necessary in order to have it included as an independent variable in the multivariate analysis.

The Analytic Model

According to the research literature cited in the previous section, physical health is causally determined by age, role losses (retirement and widowhood), income, and prior level of physical health. A generic model for identifying the relationship of exogenous variables to poor physical health (a latent or unobservable variable) was formulated and presented in figure 4-1. The model illustrates the use of six health indicators assessing physical health for 1977 and 1979. It was postulated that health in 1977 would be independently affected by five exogenous variables. Similarly, health in 1979 would be affected by the same five variables, while prior health status was taken into account. The expected structural relationships among the study variables can be formulated into an Analysis of Linear Structural Relationships (LISREL) model, a full-information maximum likelihood approach [40]. This statistical modeling technique is very appropriate to the investigation of health consequences of role losses as it allows an investigator to use latent variables and estimate (1) correlated measurement errors, (2) structural effects, and (3) correlated errors in equations.

The use of the LISREL approach requires that the following specifications be made for the model presented in figure 4-1. First, each of the five exogenous variables independently affects the latent variables. Second, since repeated measures of health indicators were used in the longitudinal study, the existence of correlated measurement errors (for example, ϵ_1 and ϵ_4, ϵ_2 and ϵ_5, and ϵ_3 and ϵ_6) needs to be examined. Third, we assumed health status was stable; therefore, an equality constraint for a given health indicator measured over time was established (for example, set $\gamma_{11} = \gamma_{42}$, $\gamma_{21} = \gamma_{52}$, and $\gamma_{31} = \gamma_{62}$). Thus, actual change (beta) in health status between 1977 and 1979 can be detected. Fourth, we followed the advice of Joreskog and Sorbom [40] to set the start value of 1

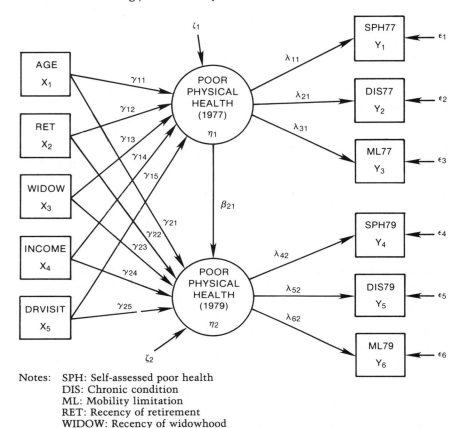

Notes: SPH: Self-assessed poor health
       DIS: Chronic condition
       ML: Mobility limitation
       RET: Recency of retirement
       WIDOW: Recency of widowhood

Figure 4–1. Generic Model for Explaining Poor Physical Health

for λ_{11} and λ_{42}. Finally, a recursive model was used since no reciprocal paths (gamma coefficients) were assumed. The effects of five exogenous variables on physical health along with other parameters were estimated. A two-tailed t-test ($\alpha = 0.5$) was performed to detect the level of significance of each parameter estimated for the model.

Results

Previous literature has clearly documented the differential effect of role loss on males and females [5, 12, 29]. Data in table 4–1 reveal that a significant difference in health status between males and females was observed for the last two waves of the longitudinal study of older adults. The sex differential in physical health measured by the three indicators

Table 4-1
Percentage Distributions of Persons Who Reported Having a
Low Level of Physical Well-Being by Health Indicators and Sex

Health Indicators	Males (N = 1,804)	Females (N = 672)	Percentage Difference between Males and Females
1977			
Perceived poor health	39.6	13.2	26.4[a]
Physical disorder	47.1	22.5	24.6[a]
Mobility limitation	33.7	0.7	33.0[a]
1979			
Perceived poor health	43.7	12.9	30.8[a]
Physical disorder	47.4	23.1	24.3[a]
Mobility limitation	38.9	0.9	38.0[a]

[a]$p < .05$.

consistently showed that the health of the male sample deteriorated at a faster rate than that of the female sample in later life.

The LISREL approach was applied to produce standardized estimates of the parameters for the model of physical health in both male and female samples. After several revisions of the study model, final results were summarized in tables 4-2 and 4-3. A goodness of fit ratio (χ^2/d.f.) of 5 or lower is considered acceptable; it is the highest tolerable level for a model fitting with a large sample [41]. When the correlated measurement errors were introduced, the degree of fitting the model to the LRHS data was substantially improved.

The Male Sample

The measurement model of physical health was first validated. The standardized factor loadings of the three indicators in 1977 and their repeated measures in 1979 showed that the presence of function-limiting conditions among males was the most dominant indicator of physical health (with factor loadings of .346 and .283 in 1977 and 1979, respectively).

Two structural equations were derived from the generic model: (1) equation 1 deals with the estimated effects of five exogenous variables on poor physical health; and (2) equation 2 includes prior health status (a latent variable) as an additional variable to estimate the causal effects of exogenous variables. The gamma coefficients under each equation show the relative importance of each exogenous variable in accounting for the variation in health status.

Table 4–2
Standardized LISREL Estimates for the Model of Poor Physical Health of Male Sample
(N = 1,804)

A. Measurement Model (Factor Loadings)[a]

Indicators	η_1 Poor Physical Health (1977)	η_2 Poor Physical Health (1979)
Y_1	.289	
Y_2	.346	
Y_3	.142	
Y_4		.236
Y_5		.283
Y_6		.116

Total coefficient of determination for Y variables is .778.

B. Structural Equation Model

Exogenous Variables	η_1 (Equation 1)	η_2 (Equation 2)
Age	.007	−.005
Recency of retirement	.068[c]	−.035
Recency of widowhood	−.083[c]	0.10
Log (income in 1975)	−.230[c]	−.067[c]
Use of physician services	.193[c]	.042
η_1 (poor physical health in 1977)		.934[c]

C. Errors (ω_i) in Equations[b]

	η_1	η_2
η_1	.901[c]	
η_2		.085

Notes: χ^2 = 91.75 with 22 degrees of freedom.
       Goodness of fit index is .991.

[a]All coefficients in the measurement model are significant at 0.01 level. The following measurement error were found to be significantly correlated: (ϵ_4, ϵ_1), (ϵ_6, ϵ_1), (ϵ_5, ϵ_2), (ϵ_6, ϵ_2), (ϵ_4, ϵ_3), (ϵ_5, ϵ_3), (ϵ_6, ϵ_3), (ϵ_6, ϵ_4).

[b]Entries on the diagonal are R^2 statistics in equations. Squared multiple correlations for equation 1 and equation 2 are .099 and .915, respectively. Total coefficient of determination for structural equations is .163.

[c]$p < .01$.

For example, in equation 1, earlier income exerted the strongest influence (– .230) on physical health although its effect was negative; the higher one's income in earlier life, the lower the probability of poor physical health in the later life.

Careful inspection of data in table 4–2 revealed several interesting findings. First, as we expected, age had a negligible effect on physical health since the study sample was relatively homogenous in its age distribution. Second, the variable "recency of retirement" had a significant positive effect on poor health. This finding implies that the longer one has retired, the greater the chance of reporting poor health. This does not mean that retirement has caused poor health since the early retirement of males might have resulted from ill health. In order to substantiate the fact that retirement did not adversely affect physical health, we examined the results associated with equation 2 and found that the relationship between the recency of retirement and physical health was not statistically significant when prior health was taken into account. Third, there was a statistically significant and negative effect of widowhood (measured by length of the event) on physical health: the more recent the widowhood, the greater the risk of poor health. When prior health was considered in equation 2, however, the relationship between widowhood and physical health vanished. This has cast some doubt on the recency effect of widowhood on the physical health of older males. Fourth, as noted before, income was the most dominant factor in accounting for the variation in physical health even though prior health was controlled in the analysis. This finding reveals the need for further exploration of mechanisms to ameliorate economic deprivation of the aged. Such mechanisms might greatly reduce their risk of poor physical health in later life.

Fifth, prior utilization of physician services had a positive effect on poor physical health status in equation 1. However, when prior health status was considered in equation 2, this relationship disappeared. There may be a spurious relationship between use of physician services and health care outcomes. Sixth, in examining equation 2, we found that there was substantial stability in rating one's physical health (β = .934). Changes in health status of older males in later life are contingent upon prior health levels. In other words, most older males' health deteriorate faster if they had poor physical health during the earlier part of their retirement. The implication for this finding is that better health should be promoted in the early stage of the aging process so that proper interventions can be instituted to either sustain or improve the health status of the aging population. Finally, the proposed model of physical health was reasonably validated in a panel design. The possibility of adding more function-assessment variables (for example, activities of daily living) to the analysis should be further explored in the interests of improving the measurement of health status.

The Female Sample

Based upon an approach similar to the one illustrated above, the female sample was analyzed by the LISREL model (table 4–3). Several major findings are worthy of discussion. First, the final model fits the data of the female sample very well, having a chi-squared value of 40.36 with 24 degrees of freedom. A substantial gain in model fitting was observed when several correlated measurement errors were introduced into the model (see note a in table 4–3). Second, the health indicators selected were relatively reliable to jointly serve as measurement instruments for the latent variables (health in 1977 and 1979). The presence of function-limiting conditions was the most dominant indicator of physical health for both periods studied.

Third, in equation 1 only two of the exogenous variables, income and use of physician services, had a statistically significant effect on poor health in 1977. None of the exogenous variables, however, had any significant influence on the physical health of females when the prior health status was considered in the second equation. The recency effect of retirement and widowhood could not be confirmed in the female sample. Fourth, females' change in physical health was not as substantial as their counterparts, as judged by the stability coefficient (beta = .788). What changes do occur are only a function of their previous health status at the early stage of their retirement.

Conclusions

Based upon a subsample of older males and females from the LRHS, a generic model for identifying the structural relationship between poor physical health and five exogenous variables was validated by the LISREL approach. The major findings of this analysis are as follows:

First, the presence of function-limiting disorders as a key indicator of physical health deserves further comment. A majority of older adults have reported chronic conditions in later life [42–44]. Yet those who are afflicted with the same condition are not necessarily limited to the same degree. This may indicate that the diagnosis-related classification has a limited utility for understanding the level of health of older adults. In other words, the presence of chronic conditions may be a necessary but not a sufficient criterion to explain the physical health status of an older

Table 4–3
**Standardized LISREL Estimates for the Model of Poor Physical Health
of Female Sample**
(N = 672)

A. *Measurement Model (Factor Loadings)*[a]

Indicators	η_1 Poor Physical Health (1977)	η_2 Poor Physical Health (1979)
Y_1	.217	
Y_2	.301	
Y_3	.158	
Y_4		.240
Y_5		.334
Y_6		.175

Total coefficient of determination for Y variables is .911.

B. *Structural Equation Model*

Exogenous Variables	η_1 (Equation 1)	η_2 (Equation 2)
Age	−.002	−.038
Recency of retirement	.039	.002
Recency of widowhood	−.038[c]	.036
Log (income in 1975)	−.297[c]	−.015
Use of physician services	.237[c]	.047
η_1 (poor physical health in 1977)		.788[c]

C. *Errors (ω_i) in Equations*[b]

	η_1	η_2
η_1	.846[c]	
η_2		.345[c]

Notes: χ^2 = 40.36 with 24 degrees of freedom.
Goodness of fit index is .989.
[a]All coefficients in the measurement model are significant at 0.01 level. The following measurement error were found to be significantly correlated. (ϵ_4, ϵ_1), (ϵ_5, ϵ_2), (ϵ_6, ϵ_3), (ϵ_6, ϵ_4), (ϵ_5, ϵ_3).
[b]Entries on the diagonal are R^2 statistics in equations. Squared multiple correlations for equation 1 and equation 2 are .154 and .655, respectively. Total coefficient of determination for structural equations is .166.
[c]$p < .01$.

population. Second, elderly persons who have a favorable level of physical health in later life are those who experienced better health at the early stage of the aging process, irrespective of major role losses, economic status, and age. It is apparent that intervention strategies need to be formulated and implemented at the period in which optimal levels of health can be achieved. This leads us to believe that the promotion of health and prevention of diseases should be a continuing process in our lives, preferably at the early stage. It would be too late to effectively intervene for any functional incapacities when one reaches advanced age.

Third, the recency of role losses, either retirement or widowhood, had a relatively negligible influence on physical health of older adults in later life. This finding has confirmed previous studies [6, 29], which found that the effect of a critical event such as widowhood may be exaggerated if an individual's prior level of health is not considered.

Fourth, the positive effect of socioeconomic status on physical health needs more attention, as this finding implies that poverty and ill health are associated: poor health in older adults cannot be changed without a concomitant improvement of economic status and health habits (directly related to life styles). Intervention strategies should be carefully formulated, along with planning for retirement, so that the health of the aged population can be greatly improved at an earlier stage.

Fifth, it is advisable, based upon the findings of the analysis, for those approaching retirement to accept the challenge to develop healthy life styles and adequate economic resources in a creative manner so that not only can one add years to one's life but also enhance life in the years to come.

Finally, a methodological note should be made with respect to the model fitting in this analysis. There are two distinct possibilities to further improve the predictive power of the generic model if future research on physical health of the old-old is to be done. First of all, investigators need to incorporate new exogenous variables into the structural equations to explain the level of physical health, such as previous levels of social well-being, measured by life satisfaction, psychological status, and other adaptation indicators. This may greatly enhance our understanding of the structural relationships between physical and social well-being of the elderly. Secondly, although the timing of role losses was found to have a negligible effect on physical health in this study, the possibility of including a perceptual variable, as measured by an individual's own perception of the critical event, should be explored in the future role loss study.

References

1. T.T.H. Wan, *Stressful Life Events, Social-Support Networks, and Gerontological Health* (Lexington, Mass.: Lexington Books, 1982).

2. I. Rosow, *Socialization to Old Age* (Berkeley, Calif.: University of California Press, 1974).

3. L.K. George, *Role Transitions in Later Life* (Monterey, Calif.: Brooks/Cole Publishing Co., 1980).

4. R.C. Atchley, "Dimensions of Widowhood in Later Life," *The Gerontologist* 15 (1975):175–178.

5. E.B. Palmore, W.P. Cleveland, J.B. Nowlin, D.R. Ramm, and I. Siegler, "Stress and Adaption in Later Life," *Journal of Gerontology* 34 (1979):841–851.

6. E.B. Palmore, G.G. Fillenbaum, and L.K. George, "Consequences of Retirement," *Journal of Gerontology* 39 (1984):109–116.

7. A.M. O'Rand, "Loss of Work Role and Subjective Health Assessment in Later Life Among Men and Married Women," in A.C. Kerckhoff (ed.), *Research in the Sociology of Education and Socialization*, Vol. 5 (Greenwich, Conn.: JAI Press, 1982).

8. T.H. Holmes and M. Masuda, "Life Change Illness Susceptibility," in B.P. Dohrenwend and B.S. Dohrenwend (eds.), *Stressful Life Events: Their Nature and Effects* (N.Y.: John Wiley & Sons, 1974).

9. R.E. Markush and R.V. Favero, "Epidemiological Assessment of Stressful Life Events, Depressed Mood, and Psychophysiological Symptoms: A Preliminary Report," in B.P. Dohrenwend and B.S. Dohrenwend (eds.), *Stressful Life Events: Their Nature and Effects* (N.Y.: John Wiley & Sons, 1974).

10. B.C. Pesznecker and J. McNeil, "Relationship Among Health Habits, Social Assets, Psychological Well-Being, Life Change, and Alterations in Health Status," *Nursing Research* 24 (1975):442–447.

11. H.S. Parnes, "From the Middle to the Later Years, Longitudinal Studies of Pre- and Post-Retirement Experiences of Men," *Research on Aging*, 3 (1981): 387–402.

12. G.F. Streib and C.J. Schneider, *Retirement in American Society: Impact and Process* (Ithaca, N.Y.: Cornell University Press, 1971).

13. W.E. Thompson, G.F. Streib, and J. Kosa, "The Effect of Retirement on Personal Adjustment: A Panel Analysis," *Journal of Gerontology* 15 (1960): 165–169.

14. J. Martin and A. Doran, "Evidence Concerning the Relationship Between Health and Retirement," *Sociological Review* 14 (1966):329–343.

15. F.M. Carp, "Housing and Living Environment of Older People," in R.H. Binstock and E. Shanas (eds.), *Handbook of Aging and the Social Sciences* (N.Y.: Van Nostrand Reinhold, 1976).

16. J. Cassel, "Physical Illness in Response to Stress," in S. Levine and N. Scotch (eds.), *Social Stress* (N.Y.: Aldine Publishing Co., 1970).

17. S.G. Haynes, A.J. McMichael, and H.A. Tyroler, "The Relationship of Normal Involuntary Retirement to Early Mortality among U.S. Rubber Workers," *Social Science and Medicine* 11 (1977):105–114.

18. W. Casscells, D. Evans, R.A. DeSilva, and J.E. Davies, "Retirement and Coronary Mortality," *The Lancet* 1(8181) (1980):1288–1289.

19. E.R. Gonzalez, "Retiring May Predispose to Fatal Heart Attack," *Journal of the American Medical Association* 243 (1980):13–14.

20. E. Shapiro and N.P. Roos, "Retired and Employed Elderly Persons: Their Utilization of Health Care Services," *The Gerontologist* 22 (1982): 187–193.

21. C.E. McConnel and F. Deljavan, "Consumption Patterns of the Retired Household," *Journal of Gerontology* 38 (1983):480–490.

22. D.J. Ekerdt, R. Bosse, and J. LoCastro, "Claims that Retirement Improves Health," *Journal of Gerontology* 38 (1983):231–236.

23. K.F. Ferraro, E. Mutran, and C.M. Barresi, "Widowhood, Health, and Friendship Support in Later Life," *Journal of Health and Social Behavior* 25 (1984):246–259.

24. G.H. Pollack, "Mourning and Adaptation," *International Journal of Psychoanalysis* 42 (1961):341–361.

25. W. Rees and S. Lutkins, "The Mortality of Bereavement," *British Medical Journal* 5 (1967):13–16.

26. D. Maddison and A. Viola, "The Health of Widows in the Year Following Bereavement," *Journal of Psychosomatic Research* 12 (1968):297–306.

27. C.M. Parkes, B. Benjamin, and R.G. Fitzgerald, "Broken Heart: A Statistical Study of Increased Mortality Among Widowers," *British Medical Journal* 1 (1969):740–743.

28. D.K. Heyman and D.T. Gianturco, "Long-term Adaptation by the Elderly to Bereavement," *Journal of Gerontology* 28 (1973):359–362.

29. F. Elwell and A.D. Maltbie-Crannell, "The Impact of Role Loss Upon Coping Resources and Life Satisfaction of the Elderly," *Journal of Gerontology* 36 (1981):223–232.

30. M. Young, B. Benjamin, and C. Wallis, "The Mortality of Widowers," *The Lancet* 2 (1963):454–456.

31. C.M. Parkes, "Effects of Bereavement on Physical and Mental Health— A Study of the Medical Records of Widows," *British Medical Journal* 2 (1964): 274–279.

32. P.J. Clayton, "Mortality and Morbidity in the First Year of Widowhood," *Archives of General Psychiatry* 30 (1974):747–750.

33. P.J. Clayton, A. Halikes, and W.L. Maurice, "The Bereavement of the Widowed," *Diseases of the Nervous System* 32 (1971):597–604.

34. T.H. Holmes and R.H. Rahe, "The Social Readjustment Rating Scale," *Journal of Psychosomatic Research* 11 (1967):213–218.

35. A. Wyler, M. Masuda, and T.H. Holmes, "Magnitude of Life Events and Seriousness of Illness," *Journal of Psychosomatic Medicine* 33 (1971):115–122.

36. R.H. Rahe, M. Meyer, M. Smith, G. Kyaer, and T.H. Holmes, "Social Stress and Illness Onset," *Journal of Psychosomatic Research* 8 (1964):35–44.

37. S. Cobb, "Social Support as a Moderator of Life Stress," *Psychosomatic Medicine* 38 (1972):300–312.

38. S.H. Beck, "Adjustment to and Satisfaction with Retirement," *Journal of Gerontology* 37 (1982):616–624.

39. L.I. Pearlin and M.A. Lieberman, "Social Sources of Emotional Distress," *Research in Community and Mental Health* 1 (1979):217–248.

40. K.G. Joreskog and D. Sorbom, *LISREL: Analysis of Linear Structural Relationships by the Method of Maximum Likelihood* (Uppsala, Sweden: Department of Statistics, University of Uppsala, 1983).

41. B. Wheaton, B. Munthen, D.F. Summers, and G.F. Summers, "Assessing Reliability and Stability in Panel Models," in D.R. Heise (ed.), *Sociological Methodology* (San Francisco: Jossey-Bass, 1977).

42. T.T.H. Wan, B.G. Odell, and D.T. Lewis, *Promoting the Well-Being of the Elderly: A Community Diagnosis* (N.Y.: Haworth Press, 1982).

43. E. Shanas, "Self-Assessment of Physical Function: White and Black Elderly of the United States," in S.G. Haynes and M. Feinleib (eds.), *Epidemiology of Aging* (Washington, D.C.: U.S. Government Printing Office, 1980).

44. L.G. Branch, "Functional Abilities of the Elderly: An Update on the Massachusetts Health Care Panel Study," in S.G. Haynes and M. Feinleib (eds.), *Epidemiology of Aging* (Washington, D.C.: U.S. Government Printing Office, 1980).

Appendix 4A

Table 4A-1
Correlation Coefficients, Means, and Standard Deviations for All Variables in the Model of Physical Health

Males[a] Females[b]	NPH77	NDIS77	NML77	NPH79	NDIS79	NML79	AGE75	RET	WIDOW	LOG (INCOME)	DRVTS
NPH77	1.000	0.539	0.321	0.489	0.392	0.022	0.073	-0.032	-0.032	-0.183	0.149
NDIS77	0.484	1.000	0.305	0.402	0.563	0.293	0.039	0.089	-0.022	-0.249	0.133
NML77	0.324	0.445	1.000	0.465	0.168	0.585	0.082	0.071	0.149	-0.139	0.130
NPH79	0.464	0.430	0.448	1.000	0.325	0.669	0.059	0.061	0.043	-0.169	0.159
NDIS79	0.401	0.594	0.370	0.410	1.000	0.187	0.009	0.043	-0.003	-0.203	0.106
NML79	0.370	0.361	0.524	0.503	0.493	1.000	0.080	0.040	0.104	-0.113	0.123
AGE75	-0.025	-0.010	0.032	-0.015	-0.050	0.006	1.000	0.095	0.083	-0.153	0.025
RET	0.032	0.047	0.054	0.050	0.034	0.043	0.058	1.000	0.065	-0.183	0.055
WIDOW	0.012	0.014	0.015	0.040	0.055	-0.017	0.112	0.026	1.000	-0.254	0.042
INCOME	-0.175	-0.229	-0.195	-0.195	-0.221	-0.136	-0.011	-0.046	-0.190	1.000	-0.026
DRVTS75	0.185	0.127	0.231	0.192	0.172	0.225	-0.214	0.054	0.029	-0.064	1.000
Males											
Mean	0.194	0.333	0.131	0.256	0.341	0.185	66.356	1.684	0.232	8.995	6.086
SD	0.396	0.471	0.337	0.437	0.474	0.389	1.706	0.914	0.665	0.797	13.479
Females											
Mean	0.132	0.225	0.074	0.129	0.231	0.085	66.388	1.771	1.126	8.464	6.558
SD	0.339	0.418	0.263	0.336	0.422	0.279	1.711	0.884	0.990	0.752	11.926

Note: Figures above the diagonal are for males and those under the diagonal are for females.
[a]N = 1,804.
[b]N = 672.

5
Social and Economic Consequences of Major Role Losses in Later Life

The notion that role loss through retirement or widowhood affects social adjustment is a durable one, and it has attracted the attention of gerontologists and social researchers for several reasons. First, evidence has been presented that the role loss experienced by retirees or widowed persons may mean the decrease in or loss of regular income and support [1-5]. Empirical research based upon both cross-sectional and longitudinal studies reveals that the causal relationship between role loss and decline in social and economic well-being has yet to be determined. Second, life-change events are not occurring randomly in later life. The concomitance of these events has significantly affected the adjustment of many individuals in the society. Such incidence is the major concern of social service practitioners. Third, the growth of the aging population indicates a need for better understanding of life transitions so that social planning can be more effectively developed to deal with the adverse effects of role losses. Fourth, negative views of role loss are consistent with the Western cultural ideology that values work and other family-related roles [6]. Finally, there is still a dearth of information about the timing of the role loss and its effect on social and economic well-being of the elderly.

The cumulative effect of role losses has not been fully demonstrated because most previous studies suffer from severe methodological faults, such as the lack of longitudinal observations of social consequences, inadequate measurements of social and economic well-being, and use of retrospective designs in collecting social data. Furthermore, there has been limited research into the social consequences of concomitant role losses such as retirement and widowhood.

This chapter will present a thorough analysis of social profiles of those who have experienced multiple role losses in later life. It will also ascertain the relationship between role losses and their effects on social and economic well-being levels of the elderly.

Related Research

Social and Economic Consequences of Retirement

Retirement may mean the loss of salary and wages. This loss of regular income requires that income be maintained through retirement benefits. It is, therefore, important to look at the economic consequences of retirement.

Morrison [7] surveyed a large sample of hourly skilled and unskilled workers with one or more years employment, aged forty-five to fifty-four years. He found that while many were anticipating financial problems in retirement, employees were not saving substantially and often held unrealistic expectations about supplementing pension benefits through earnings and accumulated savings. Statistics show slightly less than half (46%) of all workers in the private sector are covered by a pension plan wheras 90% of those employed in the public sector (federal, state or local government) are covered by pension plans [8].

Although social security benefits are a major source of retirement income for most elderly, many who have worked in employment covered by the social security program do not meet minimum requirements for retired-worker benefits. On the basis of a sample of persons near retirement age in 1973, it was found an estimated 12% of the men and 29% of the women with any covered employment from 1937 to 1973 would not be fully insured for retired-worker benefits [9]. When only those workers active after 1950 are considered, 6% of the men and 20% of the women do not qualify. As females become a larger and more stable part of the labor force, we can expect to see an even greater decrease in those not qualifying.

Inflation has had a definite impact on the elderly living on fixed incomes. They have seen their buying power decline as the cost of living rises. Some private pension plans have provided benefit increases or other forms of protection against inflation to their retired workers. In recent years, recognizing the negative effects of inflation on the purchasing power of social security benefits of retired persons in their sixties from 1970 to 1974 [10], it was found that increases in private pension benefits were not enough to prevent a decine in purchasing power for beneficiaries. However, social security benefits rose substantially more than the consumer price index in the same period. Therefore, those receiving both secondary pensions and social security benefits were able to maintain their purchasing power even in the face of high inflation.

Although almost all retirees must face a decrease in income, some are better off than others. Among 1973–74 retirees, total benefits, on the average, replaced 54% of previous earnings for those couples with retired-worker wives, and 58% for those with dependent wives [11]. The higher replacement rate for the latter group is explained mainly by the availability of dependent spouses' benefits under social security. So although earnings of the working wives contributed substantially to the couple's standard of living before retirement, the benefits for such couples are not proportionately greater after retirement. Being married also increases the likelihood of income from pensions other than social security [12], and this in turn raises the replacement rate (62% for couples with second pensions compared with 49% for those couples without) [11]. Retired married couples also have higher median incomes than nonmarried persons.

Blacks suffer the worst economic consequences in old age—a result of lifelong patterns of lower educational attainment, lower skilled jobs, and lower salaries. They were found less likely to receive income from pensions other than social security benefits or other assets [12]. They also had lower median earnings and lower median social security benefits.

Every year the earnings test penalizes a number of elderly workers for their employment by the loss of social security benefits. In 1975, one-seventh of retired workers on the social security rolls were affected by the earnings test [13]. In 1975 the earnings test provided that benefits were to be withheld at the rate of $1.00 for every $2.00 in earnings exceeding $2,520. Relatively fewer women retirees than men incurred benefit losses because relatively fewer women worked, and those who did work had lower earnings [13]. Black retired workers and those of other minority races had lower earnings than did whites.

Some researchers [14] interpret the small percentage of social security beneficiaries who have benefits suspended because of work earnings as indicating a high degree of stability in the retirement decision. However, the threat of lost benefits because of earnings can also be seen as a severe deterrent to those who would prefer some degree of employment over complete retirement.

It is apparent that some elderly choose to continue working either full- or part-time after the traditional retirement age. In a 1976 sample [12], 6 percent of couples and 3% of single persons over sixty-five had incomes comprised totally of earnings, and 35% of couples and 13% of nonmarried persons still had some earnings in combination with pension benefits. Preliminary analysis of the LRHS data [15] also shows that 12% of the study population had a shift away from retirement back into the work force. This interesting subject has not yet been studied in detail. The identification of returning workers' characteristics and the consequences they experience by re-entering the work force is worthy of further research.

Recent studies on retirement have documented little impact of retirement on social well-being [16, 17]. An analysis of data from six retirement studies found that while a slight increase in solitary activities did occur following retirement, preretirement activity level was the strongest predictor of postretirement levels [17]. Similar results were found by Glamser [18] who reported that social support networks and resources carried into retirement were directly related to postretirement attitudes. Satisfaction with leisure carried over into the retirement years [19] as demonstrated by the fact that leisure activities did not change significantly after retirement [20].

Social and Economic Consequences of Widowhood

In recent years, the research literature on widowhood has grown considerably [21–22]. Widowhood represents one of the major transition events in later life, and it has a significant influence on the well-being of older, widowed persons [23]. Previous research on widowhood has usually been focused on the adjustment of the female widowed, using data collected from a retrospective or a cross-sectional study.

Widowhood necessitates major adapations in the surviving spouse [24]. Successful re-entry into life following the loss is aided by personal, economic, and social resources. Health status, education, friendship and familial support as well as income adequacy have direct effects on the social well-being of the widowed.

Friendship networks play a dual role following the loss of a spouse. While friendship support has a direct effect on perceived health [25], it can also serve a compensatory role where increased interaction with friends makes up for the loss of spouse [26]. Ferraro and associates [25] reported no difference in the presence of friendship networks for widows and widowers. Lopata [4], however, considered widows a "socially disadvantaged" group which experienced increased social isolation. Friends avoided the bereaved because of association with death and grief, and widows themselves reduced interaction because they felt they no longer fit in. This phenomenon is especially true for those who are the first within their group to experience widowhood. Subsequent widows use their widowed friends as support networks [27].

Family members provide other essential social networks for the widowed [4, 26, 28]. Parents play an especially significant role in supporting the widowed [27]. When parents are living, support from other sources fails to mediate the effects of widowhood as well do the parents. Clayton and associates [29], on the other hand, concurred with the generally accepted belief that children are the most helpful during bereavement. During widowhood, the frequency of visits from family members was found to increase despite reductions in family size [30]. However, ethnic differences in family interaction exist, with black and Hispanic widows being more likely to receive support from family members [31]. The lower economic and poorer health statuses found for these groups may explain these differences.

Ferraro [26] in his review of the literature on the social participation of the widowed reported considerable stability in familial interaction, especially for widows. Morgan's findings [30] of continued financial support to adult children of the widowed and the negative economic impact of widowhood substantiates this finding.

Widowers were found to experience an immediate decline in interaction with parents-in-law and a long-term decrease in relations with their children [26]. Atchley [1] maintains that the economic advantages of widowers compensates for this reduction in familial interaction. This variance in economic resources offers a partial explanation of the sex difference in the adjustment to widowhood. Based upon data from their longitudinal study of men below the retirement age of sixty-five, Mott and Haurin [32] analyzed the impact of loss of spouse on widows of the deceased subjects. They reported that real income decreased following the loss of spouse. Declining income contributes to maladjustment [25] and affects health status [4], housing, and social activity [4]. Atchley [1] found that for working class females, widowhood is associated with income inadequacy which in turn is associated with low social participation and low auto use. Furthermore, depression during widowhood may be associated with financial concerns as well as loss of spouse and decreased social contacts [29].

Berardo [33] studied the role difference between males and females in their adjustment to widowhood and reported that widowers were more likely to experience interpersonal problems and social isolation than widows. This difference may be explained by the facts that widowers lack a built-in peer group of other widowers, are poorly integrated into the family or kin system, and receive less social approval for expression of emotion.

A study conducted by Atchley [1] reports that the widowed fare less well in sociopsychological consequences, with males scoring better than females on most of the well-being indicators. This finding appears to be in contrast to that of Berardo [33] and other studies [22, 34–35].

On the other hand, there are studies suggesting that the sex difference is not important in determining the level of adjustment of widowhood. For example, Arens [36], in the analysis of data collected by the Harris Study, reports that factors other than sex difference are important in accounting for the differential in adjustment among the widowed. Income and contact with friends are the most significant factors for women, while good health and club memberships are important predictors of subjective well-being for males.

In sum, based upon gender roles, research literature to date has suggested that the sex difference in role transition at widowhood may be a relevant factor in explaining the variation in adjustment or well-being of the widowed, but it is not the sole reason for asserting that more adverse effects of widowhood will be observed among males than females. Further, the long-term effect of widowhood has not been thoroughly investigated in a longitudinal study.

Concomitant Effects of Retirement and Widowhood on Social Well-Being

Retirement has been found to be related to widowhood [23]. The impact of the concomitant events can vary according to the availability of personal resources and coping mechanisms. However, resources that can be used in successful adaptation to one of these events may not be successful in dealing with both events [37].

Double economic jeopardy exists for the retired household following the death of a spouse; income already reduced by retirement may be further decreased income by widowhood. Widows are especially vulnerable because men receive higher pension incomes than women [32, 38]. The impact of the spouse's death varies depending on whether or not a lingering illness was involved since the long duration of illness can have a devastating economic effect. The medical expense associated with a lengthy illness can significantly reduce family income [32].

The occurrence of widowhood and retirement in the same time period affects areas other than economic circumstances. In a cross-sectional study of British retirement communities, Karn [39] found that both widows and widowers expressed high levels of isolation and decreased interaction with friends following the loss of spouse. Where a high level of dependency existed prior to the loss, widows experienced reduced mobility [1] and required assistance with home repairs and shopping [31].

In the initial analysis of three out of six waves of LRHS data, Wan [23] reported that retirement was significantly correlated to widowhood when the study sample was comparatively younger (fifty-eight to sixty-three years of age). Perhaps experiencing this event relatively early in life contributes to a change in life style and, consequently, to a decision to retire. Another possible interpretation is that the illness of a spouse leads to a relatively early retirement in order to be a caregiver. It is also interesting to note here that retirement or widowhood alone cannot predict that the involuntary retirement and loss of spouse in the same period will deleteriously affect one's psychological and social well-being. The present study focuses on the adjustment process of the widowed, with particular emphasis on their economic consequences—how it relates to their income status.

Methodology

Sample

Data for this analysis were obtained from the LRHS of older adults in the United States [40]. A selected sample of both males and females with complete information on the six-wave surveys was used in the present analysis. Detailed description of the study sample was presented in the previous chapter.

Because the focus of this chapter is on the social and economic well-being of older adults in later life, the 1977 and 1979 waves of the LRHS were the primary data source for identifying each individual panel member's levels of life satisfaction, happiness, and economic resources for coping with retirement and other life changes. Information about personal characteristics, social support networks, and timing of role losses (retirement and widowhood) was obtained from previous waves (particularly 1975) of the LRHS data set.

Measurement

Social well-being is a latent variable. Three indicators of social well-being employed in the analysis include (1) life satisfaction, (2) happiness, and (3) economic status. All of these variables were based on self-assessments made in 1977 and 1979. Dummy variables were constructed for satisfaction, happiness, and ability "to make ends meet with one's income." Responses of life dissatisfaction were assigned a value of 1 and others 0. Being unhappy with one's life was coded 1; otherwise it was coded 0. The inability "to make ends meet on one's income" was coded 1 and other responses were coded 0.

Five exogenous variables were used in this analysis: (1) age, (2) recency of retirement, (3) recency of widowhood, (4) income, and (5) social support networks. With the exception of social support networks, the definitions and operational measures of four variables were presented in the last chapter. A weighted composite index of social support (interaction) networks was constructed by the following procedures: (1) the frequency of interactions with spouse, children, siblings, friends, relatives, and neighbors was coded, ranging from 0 (absence of interaction) to 4 (daily contacts) for each of the social networks; and (2) an average of the sum of all five networks was then computed.

The Analytic Model

The analysis has two parts. Descriptive information about the social profiles of the study sample for this chapter was first presented to identify the differentials in social well-being levels in 1977 and 1979.

The second part of the analysis focused on a causal model of the factors affecting the level of social well-being of older males and females. The measurement model of social well-being for 1977 and 1979, and the structural relationships of five exogenous variables to the latent variables (poor social well-being in 1977 and 1979) were examined using the LISREL approach [41].

Figure 5–1 depicts a generic (hypothetical) model for the expected relationships among the study variables. The following assumptions were made for the analysis: (1) each of the exogenous variables exerted

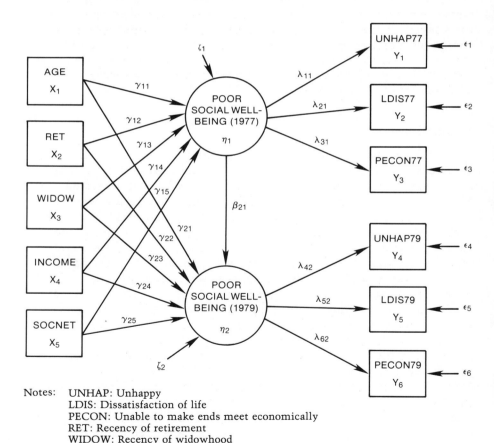

Notes: UNHAP: Unhappy
LDIS: Dissatisfaction of life
PECON: Unable to make ends meet economically
RET: Recency of retirement
WIDOW: Recency of widowhood
SOCNET: Social interaction networks

Figure 5–1. Generic Model for Explaining Poor Social Well-Being

an independent influence on the level of social well-being; (2) correlated measurement errors existed among the indicators of social well-being; (3) for each person the measurement items and their respective repeated measures of the latent variables were treated as if equal over time so that actual changes in well-being status could be estimated; and (4) estimated parameters were tested for their statistical significance, setting at the .05 level.

Results

Social Characteristics of the Study Panel of Older Males and Females

The panel (N = 2,476) selected from the LRHS was a heterogenous group with respect to social and economic characteristics, although members of the panel were all older adults (table 5–1). A majority of the panel was retired in 1975, 81 percent of the female sample and 80 percent of the male sample. The percentages of being widowed in 1975 were 7 and 55 for the male and female samples, respectively. The average age in each of the two samples was approximately 66.5 years in 1975.

Table 5–2 presents additional social profiles of the study panel in terms of their social well-being levels. In general, more than one-third of the study samples reported poor social well-being in the last three waves of LRHS. There was a steadily increasing trend of persons reporting that dissatisfaction and unhappiness. The perception of economic difficulties was relatively constant throughout the last three study periods, although one-third of the samples reported an inadequacy of income. However, no significant sex differential in social well-being levels was observed.

Table 5–1
Selected Social Characteristics of Male and Female Panel Samples in 1975

	Males	Females	Differences between Males and Females
% white	91.1	87.5	3.6
% widowed	7.0	55.2	−48.2[a]
% retired	80.0	80.7	−0.7
Mean family income	$9,536.0	$8,880.0	$656.0[a]
Average age	66.4	66.4	0
Average social networks	1.4	1.4	0

[a]p < .05.

Table 5-2
Percentage Distributions of Persons with a Low Level of Social Well-Being (SWB) by Social, Psychological, and Economic Indicators and Sex

SWB Indicators	Males (N = 1,804)	Females (N = 672)	Percentage Difference between Males and Females
1975			
Life Dissatisfied	20.4	22.4	−2.0
Unhappy	35.8	34.5	1.3
Poor economically	11.1	13.8	−2.7
1977			
Life dissatisfied	38.9	36.6	2.3
Unhappy	43.3	44.2	−0.9
Poor economically	33.5	35.2	−1.7
1979			
Life dissatisfied	39.1	36.5	2.6
Unhappy	51.9	51.0	0.9
Poor economically	33.4	34.2	0.2

The findings that older adults' perceptions about life satisfaction and happiness were deteriorating while the feeling of inadequate economic resources remained very constant in later life raised a critical issue concerning the determinants of life satisfaction in later life. The possible linkage between role loss and poor social well-being levels needs to be empirically validated.

Effects of Role Losses on Social Well-Being

The LISREL approach was applied to produce standardized estimates of the parameters for the generic model of social well-being presented in figure 5-1. When the statistical model was finalized, correlated measurement errors of social well-being indicators were included. Some interesting results were generated from the model are summarized in tables 5-3 and 5-4 for the male and female samples, respectively. Although no sex differentials in social well-being levels were noted above, the present analysis took a necessary precaution to analyze the two study samples independently in order to ensure no bias was introduced into the model since there were significant differences in the initial male and female samples.

The Male Sample. The measurement model of poor social well-being, portrayed by respondents' assessment of life satisfaction, happiness, and economic status, was first validated (table 5–3). The standardized factor loadings of the three indicators measured in both 1977 and 1979 revealed that the perception of an unhappy life was the most important indicator of poor social well-being (with factor loadings of .277 and .267 in 1977 and 1979, respectively). The six indicators of social well-being were well represented by the two latent variables, which had a reliability coefficient of .876.

Two structural equations were generated from the generic model: (1) equation 1 includes five exogenous variables—measured by age, recency of retirement and widowhood, income, and social interaction networks—to predict social well-being levels in 1977; and (2) equation 2 adds the initial social well-being (a latent variable) to the five exogenous variables, and they serve as predictors of the level of social well-being in 1979. The gamma coefficients under the equations show the relative effect of each exogenous variable on the level of well-being. For example, in equation 1 we found that both income and social interaction networks had a significantly negative influence on older males' perception of poor social well-being. The higher the income one earned, the smaller the chance one would report poor social well-being in 1977. Similarly, the stronger the social interaction (support) networks one had, the greater well-being one would experience in 1977. When the initial (1977) level of social well-being was introduced in equation 2, the only exogenous variable which remained significant was income. This implies that male adults' perception of social well-being in later life was very much conditioned by their income and prior levels of social well-being. The stability coefficient (beta = .695) shows that the level of social well-being was relatively constant. In other words, the change in social well-being of older males was contingent upon their prior status; the poorer the level of social well-being one had, the faster the decline in well-being one would experience in later life. The overall model fits well with the LRHS data, shown by a chi-square value of 57.09 with 23 degrees of freedom. Evidence has also shown that there were factors other than the five exogenous variables which might have accounted for the variation in social well-being of older males.

It is important to note here that the timing of role losses had no direct impact on social well-being of older males in later life. Two possible reasons for this are (1) the duration and timing of role losses which occur in the early stage of retirement exert no long-term influence on social well-being in later life; and (2) male adults tend to develop adap-

Table 5-3
Standardized LISREL Estimates for the Model of Poor Social Well-Being (SWB) of the Male Sample
$(N = 1,804)$

A. Measurement Model (Factor Loadings)[a]

Indicators	η_1 Poor SWB (1977)	η_2 Poor SWB (1979)
Y_1	.226	
Y_2	.277	
Y_3	.240	
Y_4		.217
Y_5		.267
Y_6		.232

Total coefficient of determination for Y variables is .876.

B. Structural Equation Model

Exogenous Variables	η_1 (Equation 1)	η_2 (Equation 2)
Age	$-.036$	$-.006$
Recency of retirement	.028	.032
Recency of widowhood	.016	$-.040$
Log (income in 1975)	$-.352^c$	$-.123^c$
Social interaction networks	$-.062^c$	$-.032$
η_1 (poor SWB in 1977)		$.695^c$

C. Errors (ω_i) in Equations[b]

	η_1	η_2
η_1	$.863^c$	
η_2		$.435^c$

Note: $\chi^2 = 57.09$ with 23 degrees of freedom.
   Goodness of fit index is .994.

[a]All coefficients in the measurement model are significant at 0.01 level. The following measurement error were found to be significantly correlated: (ϵ_4, ϵ_1), (ϵ_5, ϵ_1), (ϵ_6, ϵ_1), (ϵ_5, ϵ_2), (ϵ_4, ϵ_3) (ϵ_6, ϵ_3), (ϵ_6, ϵ_4).

[b]Entries on the diagonal are R^2 statistics in equations. Squared multiple correlations for equations 1 and 2 are .137 and .565, respectively. Total coefficient of determination for structural equations is .168.

[c]$p < .01$.

tive or coping responses to critical events—that is, widowhood and retirement—so that the compensatory activities, including social participation in both formal and informal activities, may help attenuate the adverse effect of life stress on older males.

The Female Sample. Based upon an approach similar to that presented above, the female sample was analyzed by the LISREL model (table 5–4). Major findings are presented in this section. First, the final model was validated with a chi-square value of 34.02 and 25 degrees of freedom. The model fits well with the data of the LRHS female sample. Second, older females' perception of an unhappy life was the most dominant indicator of social well-being. The three well-being indicators and their repeated measures were relatively reliable when jointly serving as measurement instruments for the latent variables (well-being in 1977 and 1979). Third, two of the five exogenous variables had statistically significant effects on the level of social well-being in 1977. However, their effects were negative; the higher the income and the more frequent the interactions with others, the smaller the chance of poor social well-being. Fourth, when the prior level of social well-being was considered, the effects of income and social interaction networks became negligible (see equation 2). However, two exogenous variables, recency of retirement and recency of widowhood, exerted a significant effect on social well-being of older females. It is possible that prior levels of social well-being were responsible for distorting the true relationship between role losses and later levels of social well-being. The significant negative effect of the timing of retirement on older females' perceptions of poor social well-being in 1979 may mean that retirement as a role loss has an immediate or short-term rather than a long-term negative impact on well-being. On the contrary, widowhood exerted a long-term rather than a short-term impact on older females' perceptions of social well-being; the longer an older female stayed widowed, the worse she perceived her social well-being.

Finally, the perceptions of social well-being remained very stable as indicated by the beta coefficient (.720). What changes did occur among older females, during the period of 1977–1979, was primarily a joint function of their initial social well-being levels and the timing of role losses experienced in later life. Data in table 5–4 showed that an older female in 1979 would be adversely affected by a combination of three conditions: (1) long-term widowhood; (2) recent retirement; and (3) perceptions of poor social well-being in 1977.

This finding confirms a synergistic effect of widowhood and retirement on self-perceptions of well-being for older females. Furthermore, the timing of these role losses is a very important factor affecting the social well-being of older females in later life.

Table 5–4
Standardized LISREL Estimates for the Model of Poor Social Well-Being (SWB) of the Female Sample
$(N = 672)$

A. Measurement Model (Factor Loadings)[a]

Indicators	η_1 Poor SWB (1977)	η_2 Poor SWB (1979)
Y_1	.202	
Y_2	.305	
Y_3	.192	
Y_4		.203
Y_5		.307
Y_6		.193

Total coefficient of determination for Y variables is .802.

B. Structural Equation Model

Exogenous Variables	η_1 (Equation 1)	η_2 (Equation 2)
Age	− .044	− .012
Recency of retirement	.033	− .072[c]
Recency of widowhood	.067	.072[c]
Log (income in 1975)	− .429[c]	− .080
Social interaction networks	− 0.095[c]	− .032
η_1 (poor SWB in 1977)		.720[c]

C. Errors (ω_i) in Equations[b]

	η_1	η_2
η_1	.782[c]	
η_2		.395[c]

Note: $\chi^2 = 34.02$ with 25 degrees of freedom.
  Goodness of fit index is .991.

[a]All coefficients in the measurement model are significant at 0.01 level. The following measurement errors were found to be significantly correlated: (ϵ_4, ϵ_1), (ϵ_5, ϵ_2), (ϵ_6, ϵ_3).

[b]Entries on the diagonal are R^2 statistics in equations. Squared multiple correlations for equations 1 and 2 are .218 and .605, respectively. Total coefficient of determination for structural equations is .169.

[c]$p < .01$.

The Structural Relationship between Physical and Social Well-Being in Later Life

The relationship between physical and social well-being was examined by a structural equation model in which four latent variables—physical health (PH) and social well-being (SWB) for 1977 and 1979—were incorporated into a recursive model. The following assumptions were made: (1) each latent variable was determined by its prior level of well-being; (2) social well-being was affected by physical health; and (3) each of the latent variables was affected by five exogenous variables. There is a plausible reciprocity between physical and social well-being variables as they may affect each other in a theoretical sense. In other words, social well-being may be affected by physical health, while physical health may also be affected by social well-being. Several attempts to analyze the LISREL results yielded a final model, presented in figure 5-2, in which no lagged effect of SWB77 on PH79 or PH77 on SWB79 was established. This model offers a better fitting to the LRHS data than other (cross-lagged) models.

Table 5–5 presents a summary of LISREL results for the male sample. Several major findings are worthy of note here. First, the goodness of fit of the proposed generic model was reasonably validated by incorporating the correlated measurement errors of the four latent variables. The direct causal effect of physical health (η_1) on social well-being (η_2) was statistically significant in 1977. This means the higher the level of physical well-being, the better the perception of social well-being. A similar result was found for the relationship between the two latent variables in 1979. The physical and social well-being levels were relatively stable as indicated by strong positive beta coefficients linking each of the same latent variables between 1977 and 1979. Second, the exogenous variables, measured in 1975, exerted a strong direct effect on physical and social well-being in 1977 but not in 1979. Again, as found in previous sections, no effect of retirement and widowhood on older males' social well-being was found when prior health and social well-being were taken into account in the analysis. Third, income was the only exogenous variable that consistently related to the well-being of males. Fourth, the overall fitness of the generic model (figure 5-2) was substantially improved when the prior health level was added to the original model presented in figure 5-1. Data appear to confirm the fact that perceptions of social well-being in later life were greatly enhanced if one had a better physical, as well as social, well-being in the earlier period of the retirement age.

By using a similar approach, the structural relationship between physical health and social well-being of the female sample (table 5–6)

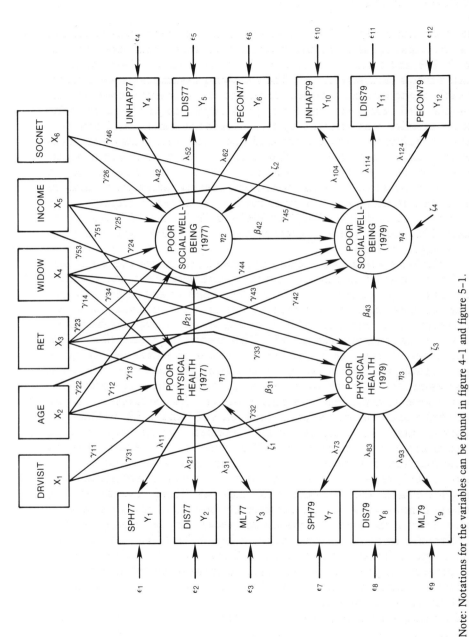

Note: Notations for the variables can be found in figure 4–1 and figure 5–1.

Figure 5–2. A Model for Explaining the Structural Relationship Between Physical Health and Social Well-Being For Older Adults in Later Life

Table 5-5
Standardized LISREL Estimates for the Model of Physical Health (PH) and Social Well-Being (SWB) of the Male Sample
$(N = 1,804)$

A. Measurement Model (Factor Loadings)[a]

Indicators	η_1 Poor PH (1977)	η_2 Poor SWB (1979)	η_3 Poor PH (1977)	η_4 Poor SWB (1979)
Y_1	.293			
Y_2	.324			
Y_3	.155			
Y_4		.233		
Y_5		.289		
Y_6		.215		
Y_7			.252	
Y_8			.279	
Y_9			.133	
Y_{10}				.207
Y_{11}				.257
Y_{12}				.191

Total coefficient of determination for Y variables is 0.939.

B. Structural Equation Model

Exogenous Variables	η_1 (Equation 1)	η_2 (Equation 2)	η_3 (Equation 3)	η_4 (Equation 4)
Doctor visits (X_1)	.201	0	.041	0
Age (X_2)	.012	$-.044^c$	$-.006$	$-.008$
Retirement (X_3)	$.068^d$	$-.011$	$-.035$	.034
Widowhood (X_4)	$-.075^c$	.048	$-.002$	$-.045^c$
Income (X_5)	$-.227^d$	$-.240^d$	$-.067^d$	$-.148^d$
Social networks (X_6)	0	$-.046^c$	0	$-.037$
η_1 (PH77)		$.516^d$	$-.905^d$	
η_2 (SWB77)				$.631^d$
η_3 (PH79)				$.103^c$

C. Errors (ω_1) in Equations[b]

	η_1	η_2	η_3	η_4
1	$.899^d$			
2		$.610^d$		
3			$.141^d$	
4			$.173^d$	$.380^d$

Note: $\chi^2 = 379.4$ with 92 degrees of freedom. Goodness of fit index $= .977$.

[a]All coefficients in the measurement model are significant at 0.01 level. The following measurement errors were found to be significantly correlated: (ϵ_1, ϵ_7), (ϵ_2, ϵ_8), (ϵ_3, ϵ_9), $(\epsilon_4, \epsilon_{10})$, $(\epsilon_5, \epsilon_{11})$, $(\epsilon_6, \epsilon_{12})$, (ϵ_1, ϵ_9), (ϵ_3, ϵ_9), (ϵ_4, ϵ_6), (ϵ_7, ϵ_9), $(\epsilon_{\cdot}, \epsilon_{12})$.

[b]Entries on the diagonal are R^2 statistics in equations. Squared multiple correlations for four structural equations are 0.101, 0.390, 0.859, and 0.620, respectively.

[c]$p < .05$.

[d]$p < .01$.

Table 5-6
Standardized LISREL Estimates for the Model of Physical Health (PH) and Social Well-Being (SWB) of the Female Sample
(N = 672)

A. Measurement Model (Factor Loadings)[a]

Indicators	η_1 Poor PH (1977)	η_2 Poor SWB (1977)	η_3 Poor PH (1979)	η_4 Poor SWB (1979)
Y_1	.213			
Y_2	.250			
Y_3	.167			
Y_4		.219		
Y_5		.290		
Y_6		.201		
Y_7			.233	
Y_8			.273	
Y_9			.182	
Y_{10}				.209
Y_{11}				.277
Y_{12}				.192

Total coefficient of determination for Y variables is 0.941.

B. Structural Equation Model

Exogenous Variables	η_1 (Equation 1)	η_2 (Equation 2)	η_3 (Equation 3)	η_4 (Equation 4)
Doctor visits (X_1)	.275	.000	.007	.000
Age (X_2)	.008	−.057	−.032	−.010
Retirement (X_3)	.043	.021	−.004	−.077[c]
Widowhood (X_4)	−.042	.072	.035	.080[c]
Income (X_5)	−.308[d]	−.342[d]	.053	−.090[c]
Social networks (X_6)	.000	−.064	.000	−.030
η_1 (PH77)		.273[c]	.999[d]	
η_2 (SWB77)				.680[d]
η_3 (PH79)				.091

C. Errors (ω_1) in Equations[b]

	η_1	η_2	η_3	η_4
1	.819[d]			
2		.120	.656[d]	
3			.027	
4			.083[c]	.357[c]

Note: χ^2 = 156.89 with 91 degrees of freedom. Goodness of fit index = .975.

[a]All coefficients in the measurement model are significant at 0.01 level. The following measurement errors were found to be significantly correlated: (ϵ_1, ϵ_7), (ϵ_2, ϵ_8), (ϵ_3, ϵ_9), $(\epsilon_4, \epsilon_{10})$, $(\epsilon_5, \epsilon_{11})$, $(\epsilon_6, \epsilon_{12})$, (ϵ_1, ϵ_2), (ϵ_8, ϵ_9).

[b]Entries on the diagonal are R^2 statistics in equations. Squared multiple correlations for four structural equations are 0.182, 0.344, 0.973, and 0.643, respectively.

[c]$p < .05$.

[d]$p < .01$.

was analyzed. Results of this analysis were quite similar to those of the male sample, although significant differences were found in the identification of the direct causal impact of exogenous variables on social well-being. For instance, when the initial health and social well-being dimensions were considered, the recency effect of retirement and the latency effect of widowhood on older females' social well-being in 1979 were statistically significant. The relationship between the two latent variables, physical health and social well-being, was significantly related in 1977 but not in 1979. In general, the results in table 5–6 showed that the generic model, with necessary revisions, fit the female data well.

Conclusions

The use of LISREL approach allows us to tease out the causal linkage between major role losses and social well-being for both the male and female study samples. We found that the timing of retirement and widowhood exerted no direct impact on the social well-being of older males when the prior level of social well-being and other personal characteristics such as age, income, and social support networks were controlled. A distinct difference was observed in the female sample, however. Among older females there appeared to be a recency effect of retirement and a latency effect of widowhood on perceptions of social well-being when other exogenous variables and the prior level of social well-being were held constant in the analysis. This gender difference in perceptions of social well-being, as related to role losses and other personal attributes of older adults, can be interpreted in two ways. First, older males may be less sensitive to critical events such as retirement and widowhood than are older females. It is quite possible that older males' role losses could be compensated for or replaced by other social activities, either with formal or informal participation. Furthermore, the most dominant force in perceptions of social well-being is an individual's prior level of well-being. For older males, the change in social well-being in later life is contingent upon their previous perceptions of their social, psychological, and economic circumstances, not the role loss experienced. Second, longitudinal studies on role loss have several well-recognized sources of bias. For instance, in the present analysis the average age of both male and female samples combined was approximately seventy-one years in 1979. The age and sex differential in mortality may have affected the results since males who survived in advanced age were a very selective group of individuals. The timing of role losses and the magnitude of their effects on the perceptions of well-being of older adults warrant further study since it may imply that genetic, constitutional, and social perceptual factors associated with gender may be attributed to the differential susceptibility to having poor perceptions of social well-being.

According to previous studies [23, 42], the availability and use of coping resources and responses dealing with life changes may help attenuate the adverse effect of role loss. Future research must include the coping mechanisms as an intervening variable in the investigation of the structural relationship between role losses and poor perceptions of social well-being.

From a programmatic standpoint, the findings from this analysis suggest that early interventions in life satisfaction and economic resources can promote the well-being of the aged in later life. There is every reason to expect that among the young-old, the coping mechanisms for handling life stress can be easily fortified by adopting preventive and social planning strategies, such as the use of supportive social networks, preretirement planning and education, and financial planning. The early prevention of physical illness and poor perceptions of social well-being plays a pivotal role in the development of successful aging. Only with a concerted effort toward striving after happiness will the negative experiences of role losses recede in their influence on the well-being of the aged.

Finally, our findings substantiate the fact that investigators who assume a direct linear relationship between role losses and well-being are liable to oversimplify the complex phenomenon of aging and health. Greater payoffs in aging research will be gained from consideration of the life-change events, particularly those related to retirement and widowhood, as a part of the normal aging process. Thus, stronger emphasis can be placed on promoting the well-being of the elderly in the preretirement rather than the retirement stage [43, 44].

References

1. R.C. Atchley, "Dimensions of Widowhood in Later Life," *The Gerontologist* 15 (1975):175–178.

2. A. Foner and K. Schwab, *Aging and Retirement* (Monterey, Calif.: Brooks/Cole Publishing Co., 1980).

3. J. Schulz, *The Economics of Aging* (Belmont, Calif.: Wadsworth Publishing Co., 1980).

4. H.Z. Lopata, "Widows as a Minority Group," *The Gerontologist* 11 (1971):67–77.

5. L.A. Morgan, "Widows and Widowers: Changing Family Support Systems," unpublished manuscript.

6. D.J. Ekerdt, R. Bosse, and J. LoCastro, "Claims that Retirement Improves Health," *Journal of Gerontology* 38 (1983):231–236.

7. M.H. Morrison, "Planning for Income Adequacy in Retirement: The Expectations of Current Workers," *The Gerontologist* 16 (1976):538–543.

8. F.P. King, "The Future of Private and Public Employee Pension," in B.R. Herzog (ed.), *Aging and Income* (N.Y., Human Sciences Press, 1978).

9. L.B. Mallan and D. Cox, "Older Workers Uninsured for Retired-Worker Benefits," *Social Security Bulletin*, 41 (1978):3–11.

10. G.B. Thompson, "Impact of Inflation on Private Pensions of Retirees, 1970–74: Findings from the Retirement History Study," *Social Security Bulletin* 41 (1978):16–26.

11. A. Fox, "Earnings Replacement Issues of Retired Couples: Findings from the Retirement History Study," *Social Security Bulletin* 42 (1979):17–39.

12. S. Grad and K. Foster, "Income of the Population Aged 55 and Older, 1976," *Social Security Bulletin* 42 (1979):16–32.

13. B.A. Lingg, "Beneficiaries Affected by the Annual Earnings Test in 1975," *Social Security Bulletin* 41 (1978):12–24.

14. S. Grad, "New Retirees and the Stability of the Retirement Decision," *Social Security Bulletin* 40 (1977):3–12.

15. J. Murray, "Subjective Retirement," *Social Security Bulletin* 42 (1979): 20–25.

16. W.E. Thompson, G.F. Streib, and J. Kosa, "The Effect of Retirement on Personal Adjustment: A Panel Analysis," *Journal of Gerontology* 15 (1960): 165–169.

17. E.B. Palmore, G.G. Fillenbaum, and L.K. George, "Consequences of Retirement," *Journal of Gerontology* 39 (1984):109–116.

18. F.D. Glamser, "Determinants of a Positive Attitude Toward Retirement," *Journal of Gerontology* 31 (1976):104–107.

19. A.I. Weiner and S.L. Hunt, "Retirees' Perceptions of Work and Leisure Meanings," *The Gerontologist* 21 (1981):444–446.

20. R. Bosse and D.J. Ekerdt, "Change in Self-Perception of Leisure Activities with Retirement," *The Gerontologist* 21 (1981):650–654.

21. C.J. Barrett, "Women on Widowhood," *Signs* 2 (1977):856–868.

22. S.R. Hiltz, "Widowhood: A Roleless Role," *Marriage and Family Review* 1 (1978):3–10.

23. T.T.H. Wan, *Stressful Life Events, Social-Support Networks, and Gerontological Health: A Prospective Study* (Lexington, Mass.: Lexington Books, 1982).

24. L.K. George, *Role Transitions in Later Life* (Monterey, Calif.: Brooks/ Cole Publishing Co., 1980).

25. K.F. Ferraro, E. Mutran, and C.M. Barresi, "Widowhood, Health, and Friendship Support in Later Life," *Journal of Health and Social Behavior* 25 (1984):246–259.

26. K.F. Ferraro, "Widowhood and Social Participation in Later Life: Isolation or Compensation?," *Research on Aging* 6 (1984):451–468.

27. E.A. Bankoff, "Aged Parents and Their Widowed Daughters: A Support Relationship," *Journal of Gerontology* 38 (1983):226–230.

28. D.K. Heyman and D.T. Gianturco, "Long-term Adaptation by the Elderly to Bereavement," *Journal of Gerontology* 28 (1973):359–362.

29. P.J. Clayton, J.A. Halikes, and W.L. Maurice, "The Bereavement of the Widowed," *Diseases of the Nervous System* 32 (1971):597–604.

30. L.A. Morgan, "Intergenerational Economic Assistance to Children: The Case of Widows and Widowers," *Journal of Gerontology* 38 (1983):725–731.

31. A.O. Pelham and W.F. Clark, "Widowhood Among Low-income Ethnic Minorities in California." *Paper presented at the 111th Annual Meeting of the American Public Health Association, Dallas, November, 1983.*

32. *F.L. Mott and R.J. Haurin, "The Impact of Health Problems and Mortality on Family Well-Being," in H.S. Parnes (ed.), Work and Retirement: A Longitudinal Study of Men* (Cambridge, Mass.: MIT Press, 1981).

33. F.M. Berardo, "Survivorship and Social Isolation: The Case of the Widower," *Family Coordinator* 19 (1970):11–25.

34. I.O. Glick, R.S. Weiss, and C.M. Parkes, *The First Year of Bereavement* (N.Y.: John Wiley & Sons, 1974).

35. E.W. Bock and I.L. Webber, "Suicide Among the Elderly: Isolating Widowhood and Mitigating Alternatives," *Journal of Marriage and the Family* 34 (1972):24–31.

36. D.A. Arens, "Widowhood and Well-Being: An Interpretation of Sex Differences," Paper presented at the 32nd Annual Meeting of the Gerontological Society, Washington, D.C., 1979.

37. E.B. Palmore, C. William, J.B. Nowlin, D.F. Ramm, and I. Siegler, "Stress and Adaption in Later Life," *Journal of Gerontology* 34 (1979):841–851.

38. A.M. O'Rand, "Loss of Work Role and Subjective Health Assessment in Later Life Among Men and Married Women," in A.C. Kerckhoff (ed.), *Research in the Sociology of Education and Socialization*, Vol. 5 (Greenwich, Conn.: JAI Press, 1982).

39. V. Karn, "Retirement Resorts in Britain—Successes and Failures," *The Gerontologist* 20 (1980):331–341.

40. L.M. Irelan, "Retirement History Study: Introduction," *Social Security Bulletin* 35 (1972):24–33.

41. K.G. Joreskog, and D. Sorbom, *LISREL: Analysis of Linear Structural Relationships by the Method of Maximum Likelihood* (Uppsala, Sweden: Department of Statistics, University of Uppsala, 1983).

42. S.H. Beck, "Adjustment to and Satisfaction with Retirement," *Journal of Gerontology* 37 (1982):616–624.

43. F.D. Glamser, "The Impact of Pre-retirement Programs on the Retirement Experience," *Journal of Gerontology* 36 (1981):244–250.

44. E. Mutran and D.C. Reitzes, "Intergenerational Support Activities and Well-Being," *American Sociological Review* 49 (1984):117–130.

Appendix 5A

Table 5A-1
Correlation Coefficients, Means, and Standard Deviations for All Variables in the Model of Social Well-Being

Males[a] / Females[b]	UNHAP77	LDIS77	ECON77	UNHAP79	LDIS79	ECON79	AGE75	RET	WIDOW	LOG (INCOME)	WSNET-WRK
UNHAP77	1.000	0.387	0.263	0.400	0.245	0.198	0.011	0.072	0.079	-0.218	-0.089
LDIS77	0.412	1.000	0.450	0.272	0.408	0.304	0.010	0.046	0.042	-0.265	-0.095
ECON77	0.261	0.368	1.000	0.209	0.275	0.424	0.022	0.057	0.073	-0.274	-0.028
UNHAP79	0.515	0.305	0.240	1.000	0.305	0.249	0.019	0.051	-0.004	-0.187	-0.099
LDIS79	0.287	0.409	0.247	0.347	1.000	0.337	0.028	0.069	0.025	-0.219	-0.041
ECON79	0.208	0.295	0.444	0.282	0.336	1.000	0.011	0.078	0.074	-0.295	-0.061
AGE75	-0.094	0.021	-0.017	-0.060	0.016	-0.026	1.000	0.095	0.083	-0.153	-0.017
RET	0.007	0.007	0.083	-0.022	-0.014	-0.025	0.058	1.000	0.065	-0.183	0.023
WIDOW	0.051	0.090	0.089	0.126	0.097	0.077	0.112	-0.026	1.000	-0.254	0.008
INCOME	-0.218	-0.296	-0.309	-0.209	-0.226	-0.294	-0.011	-0.046	-0.190	1.000	0.107
WSNETWRK	-0.084	-0.076	-0.077	-0.057	-0.070	-0.096	-0.024	0.036	0.127	0.105	1.000
Males											
Mean	0.186	0.251	0.129	0.188	0.275	0.137	66.356	1.684	0.232	8.995	1.395
SD	0.389	0.433	0.335	0.391	0.519	0.344	1.706	0.914	0.665	0.797	0.545
Females											
Mean	0.159	0.265	0.144	0.158	0.271	0.135	66.388	1.771	1.126	8.464	1.395
SD	0.366	0.442	0.352	0.365	0.510	0.342	1.711	0.884	0.990	0.752	0.568

Note: Figures above the diagonal are for males and those below the diagonal are for females.
[a] N = 1,804.
[b] N = 672.

6
Retirement Attitudes of Married Couples in Later Life

A substantial body of previous research examines the consequences of retirement on the health and well-being of older people. Most of this research has focused on the reactions to retirement experienced by individuals, almost exclusively men. Studies of women's retirement experiences are still scarce and studies of how couples adjust to retirement are even more scarce. Given that (1) more American women are working than ever before and (2) larger numbers of male retirees are still married and residing with their spouses, research on how couples adjust to retirement is needed. Atchley [1], speaking for an eminent panel of researchers and administrators, notes the lack of attention given to the effect of retirement on couples and raises several research questions for subsequent investigation. The present research focuses on one of the questions assigned high priority by Atchley [1]: "How do variations in the retirement status of the husband and wife affect the couple's reaction to retirement?"

To answer this question we first turn to a brief consideration of the literature describing how retirement affects attitudes toward retirement among individuals and then consider the research examining couples. While a number of studies have examined the relationship between retirement and morale [2–5], the focus on this review is on attitudes toward retirement per se.

Related Research

Retirement Attitudes of Individuals

Most research on the retirement attitudes of individuals during the last two decades reports overall satisfaction [6–7]. In one of the early longitudinal studies on the subject, Streib and Schneider [8] report that both men and women are more likely to feel they should retire as they age.

Coauthored with Kenneth F. Ferraro.

Moreover, their study indicates that most retirees are relatively satisfied with retirement. Cross-sectional studies tend to report similar results. A ten-year longitudinal study of older men in Iowa by Goudy and associates [9] confirms this general finding but indicates that the degree of change in retirement attitudes is slight. Recently, Palmore and associates [10] used a national longitudinal survey that also shows that retirement creates more favorable attitudes toward retirement.

In short, though some apprehension just prior to retirement is not uncommon, most Americans hold favorable views of retirement. More importantly, most studies indicate that both men and women favor retirement more once they have experienced it.

Retirement Attitudes of Couples

While several studies have either tangentially considered spouses [11] or family relations [8, 12], only two studies focus on the couple's reactions to retirement. Both of these studies are based on cross-sectional data.

Lipman [13] studied 100 older couples in the Miami metropolitan area and focused on morale and marital satisfaction. While the variables examined do not coincide with those emphasized in the present research, two of his findings are noteworthy. First, whereas ". . . the wife is forced to adjust to her readjusting husband," it is incorrect to assume that her role conceptions and attitudes will remain unchanged. Rather, the husband-wife dyad is a social system, although small in number, which implies that a change in one person is most likely to be associated with a change in the other. Second, Lipman suggests that ". . . role differentiation by sex is reduced with increased age and retirement." Such a statement is proffered after noting the increased propensity of retired men to offer household assistance.

The other study of couples' attitudes toward retirement was conducted by Kerckhoff [14] on 198 white couples from the Piedmont region of North Carolina and Virginia. Of these couples, 108 were retired after the age of sixty and before the age of seventy; the remaining 90 couples were defined as preretirees. While the questions asked of both groups were not identical, it appears that retired couples were slightly more positive about retirement than preretired couples, especially among the men. Women tended to be more stable in their attitudes while men showed more variability over time. Using cross-sectional data, Kerckhoff [14] infers that men are favorable toward retirement before it occurs and initially favorable after retirement, but eventually become more negative—even more negative than their wives. Kerckhoff's work also indicates that the retirement attitudes of couples are substantially influenced by their position in the stratification of society (that is, a positive monotonic relationship between social class ranking and satisfaction with retirement).

Research Questions

Two salient research questions can be drawn from the review of the literature. The first, mentioned earlier in the introduction, deals with the *change* in retirement attitudes of couples. According to Atchley [1], understanding change in the retirement attitudes of couples is crucial in advancing this body of knowledge. Lipman [13] suggests that wives are just as likely as their husbands to manifest change while Kerckhoff [14] reports that wives' retirement attitudes are more stable than their husbands' retirement attitudes. The present study is designed with longitudinal data in order to more directly deal with assessments of change.

The second question deals with the degree of attitude *convergence* between husband and wife. If their attitudes toward retirement change differentially, then one can assume that their attitudes are not wholly convergent. As Rubin [15] and Bernard [16] have noted, we too often assume attitudinal and perceptual convergence in marriage. Rather, according to these authors, we can safely assume that the perceptual reality of any marriage is unique to husband and wife. In Bernard's [16] words, there are "his" and "her" marriages—really two marriages in one.

The present research is designed to examine both attitudinal *convergence* and *change* among couples experiencing retirement. A causal model for explaining the retirement attitudes of married couples is developed and tested with data from a national longitudinal survey.

Methodology

Sample

Data for this research came from the LRHS of older adults in the United States [17]. The original sample of 1969 LRHS consisted of 11,153 persons, aged fifty-eight to sixty-three, who were interviewed to examine the retirement transition. These individuals constituted a sample drawn by stratified random cluster sampling procedures as used in the Current Population Survey of the Bureau of the Census. Panel members were interviewed at two-year intervals from 1969 to 1979 on selected topics. While no attitudinal information was available in the earlier issues of the LRHS, the present research makes use of two recent waves (1977 and 1979) to examine the retirement attitudes of married couples.

The 1977 and 1979 waves contained 7,079 and 6,270 cases, respectively. The present research examines a purposive subsample of the LRHS—all those men who were married to the same person during the initial (1969) and 1979 surveys. The wives of these men were also interviewed regarding a number of issues, including their work experience and attitudes toward retirement. Excluded from the analysis were all men (and their wives) who had never worked or who were completely disabled in 1969. The number of cases for which there is complete information on the variables selected is 1,409.

The retirement attitudes of these men and women cannot simply be compared to men and women in general. Whereas the focus of this study is on couples, the men and women examined here may vary in their attitudes from men and women who are widowed, separated, divorced, or never married. Also, some caution is needed in attempting to generalize results from this research to the population of older couples in the United States. Specifically, individuals who suffered high levels of disability and were unable to work, in 1969 or before, have been excluded. We are interested in the typical attitudes toward retirement among older workers, not those forced to retire because of failing health. The consequence of this selection factor is probably more favorable attitudes toward retirement.

With these cautions in mind, the sample is one that can significantly contribute to our understanding of married couples' retirement attitudes. Since it is a national sample, it is not constrained by regional variations. More importantly it provides multiple indicators of retirement attitudes over time. Whereas previous research on this subject is based on cross-sectional samples which are constrained by region, race, and social class, the LRHS provides data that can better help us understand the *process* of adjusting to retirement among the majority of America's older couples.

One other methodological concern regards how the personal interviews were conducted. Specifically, couples were interviewed simultaneously in their own household. Whereas the present research is concerned with the degree of convergence in retirement attitudes between husband and wife, simultaneous interviewing may mean that the responses are overestimates of the degree of convergence. Being interviewed in the presence of one's spouse may foster similarity in attitudes. On the other hand, it could be argued that simultaneous interviewing may constrain couples to be more truthful about their attitudes, whether they are convergent or divergent. While there is no wholly acceptable solution to this problem because of the study design, we were initially more concerned with overestimating convergence. This concern remains but is not nearly as important after studying the intercorrelations among the attitudes of husbands and wives.

Measurement

Both husbands and wives were asked three identical questions about retirement during 1977 and 1979 interviews. For most of the analysis these questions were used to create two latent variables reflecting attitudes toward retirement for each survey period. A description of the questions and their response categories may be found in tables 6-1 and 6-2.

A number of exogenous variables were used in the analysis. Four dummy variables were created for the retirement status of the husbands and wives at both interviews (scored 0 not retired; 1 retired). Household income was measured in 23 categories ranging from 1 (under $1,000) to 23 ($30,000 and over). Given the findings of previous research, variables were also included on health and social functioning. Health was evaluated by a functional status rating for each spouse, ranging from 0 (not limited) to 3 (severely limited). The measure of social functioning is a global assessment of the husband's satisfaction with the level of activities in which he is currently involved. This variable is referred to as activity dissatisfaction and ranges from 1 (more than satisfactory) to 4 (very unsatisfactory).

Analysis

The analysis of descriptive data is presented to examine the retirement attitudes of the husbands and wives separately. These retirement attitudes are investigated in their relationship to retirement status at each interview. Then, causal analysis is performed to focus on the factors influencing the retirement attitudes of older husbands and wives and the like relationship between their attitudes.

Figure 6-1 presents a hypothetical model for the expected relationships using the LISREL approach [18]. Before discussing results, a few comments on this figure should aid understanding of the analytic strategy. The model illustrates the use of the twelve items assessing retirement attitudes for the creation of four latent variables. The procedure selected for analysis allows us to examine correlated measurement errors among the items. This is important with longitudinal data since frequently there are time-dependent error structures in models of this sort (for example, ϵ_1 and ϵ_7; see Wheaton and associates [19] for a discussion of these issues). In addition, we followed the advice of Sorbom [20]

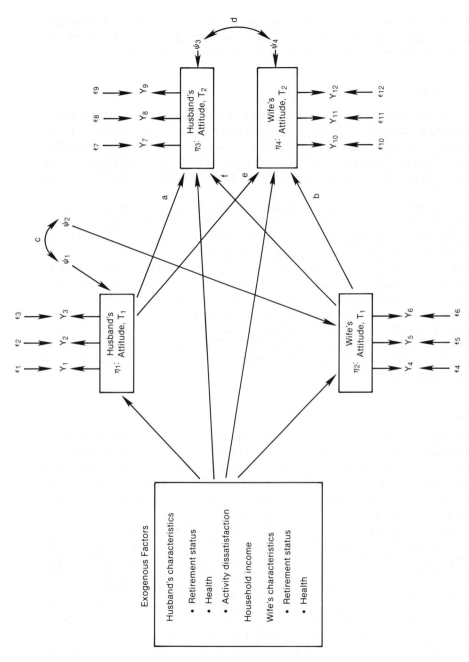

Figure 6–1. Hypothetical Model to Estimate the Retirement Attitudes of Married Couples in Later Life

to constrain the latent variables (for each person) to be equal over time so as to actually measure change in either the husband's or the wife's attitudes.

The relationships among the latent variables depicted in figure 1 have been specified for several reasons. First, a stability coefficient for both husbands (a) and wives (b) is identified between the two time periods. These coefficients allow for a comparison of the spouse's degree of stability or change in their retirement attitudes over time. Second, preliminary analysis of reciprocal paths between the attitudes of husbands and wives at each time period were not significant. Therefore, we have assumed these variables are not causally related, but have correlated errors (c at time 1 and d at time 2). These effects can be interpreted as partial correlations, the net of the effects of the exogenous variables, and may be construed as representing (residual) convergence between the attitudes of the spouses. Finally, these effects plus cross-lagged regression coefficients (e,f,) are generally the important parameters to be estimated in the analysis of longitudinal data. Examples which strongly influenced the specification of this model include the work of Campbell and Mutran [21] and Joreskog [22].

Results

Tables 6–1 and 6–2 present frequency distributions of attitudes toward retirement and percentage distributions of these attitudes by retirement status for both years among men and women respectively. First, most of the men in this sample are retired in 1977 with only a slight increase by 1979. Second, most of the men seem quite favorable toward retirement as judged by the frequency distributions. Third, retired men are more favorable toward retirement than those still employed.

The results in table 6–2 for women show some similar patterns, but the major difference is that substantially fewer women are retired. Another important difference is that the attitudes of women have smaller variance than those of the men, especially on items 1 and 3.

Table 6–3 presents the standardized LISREL estimates for the model of the retirement attitudes of married couples. This model is the one selected after more than a dozen different models were estimated. Some of the earlier models examined other variables, including the health of both husband and wife for predicting retirement attitudes. Health status showed no significant effects, probably because of the sample selection factor mentioned earlier, and was deleted from further analysis. The χ^2/d.f. ratio for the model is approximately five—the highest tolerable level for models with large samples [19]. More important than this is the

Table 6-1
Percentage Distributions of Attitudes toward Retirement by
Retirement Status Among Men

	1977			1979		
Variable	Percent Retired	Base Number	X^2	Percent Retired	Base Number	X^2
All men	91.34	1,409		93.12	1,409	
Retirement is a pleasant time of life (Y_1 in 1977, Y_7 in 1979)						
Strongly agree	97.13	244		98.10	263	
Agree	92.50	840		94.58	830	
Disagree	83.86	285		84.56	272	
Strongly disagree	85.00	40	33.97[a]	88.64	44	45.40[a]
People are foolish who don't retire when they can (Y_2 in 1977, Y_8 in 1979)						
Strongly agree	97.10	207		97.42	233	
Agree	95.75	777		96.26	721	
Disagree	82.44	393		85.75	393	
Strongly disagree	56.25	32	116.98[a]	79.41	34	61.53[a]
Older workers should retire to give younger ones a chance (Y_3 in 1977, Y_9 in 1979)						
Strongly agree	98.48	198		96.60	206	
Agree	94.60	834	95.58		792	
Disagree	81.01	337		86.83	372	
Strongly disagree	75.00	40	83.00[a]	84.62	39	38.75[a]

[a] $p < .001$.

relative fit and degree of improvement in the chi-square value per degree of freedom [22]. Some of our initial models had ratios greater than twelve. Significant improvements in model fit were made by estimating correlated measurement errors as indicated in note a of the table.

Section A of table 6-3 indicates that all of the items significantly define the constructs and displays the standardized factor loadings of the four variables. Section B presents the results of the structural equation model. The first equation (in column 1) represents the effects of the exogenous characteristics on the husbands' retirement attitudes. Recalling that the low values on the retirement items represent more favorable attitudes, it can be seen that retirement is associated with more favorable attitudes. More favorable attitudes among husbands at time

Table 6-2
Percentage Distributions of Attitudes toward Retirement by Retirement Status among Women

Variable	1977			1979		
	Percent Retired	Base Number	X^2	Percent Retired	Base Number	X^2
All women	64.09	1,409		69.98	1,409	
Retirement is a pleasant time of life (Y_4 in 1977, Y_{10} in 1979)						
Strongly agree	77.29	207		84.36	211	
Agree	63.70	967		70.21	940	
Disagree	53.81	223		59.23	233	
Strongly disagree	58.33	12	26.154[a]	40.00	25	44.31[a]
People are foolish who don't retire when they can (Y_5 in 1977, Y_{11} in 1979)						
Strongly agree	75.48	208		84.73	203	
Agree	66.63	863		71.05	836	
Disagree	50.91	330		60.22	357	
Strongly disagree	37.50	8	41.51[a]	38.46	13	45.80[a]
Older workers should retire to give younger ones a chance (Y_6 in 1977, Y_{12} in 1979)						
Strongly agree	74.21	159		78.85	156	
Agree	66.19	911		73.42	839	
Disagree	53.25	323		60.21	387	
Strongly disagree	62.50	16	25.33[a]	51.85	27	32.38[a]

[a]$p < .001$.

one are also noted for those who are more satisfied with their level of activity and whose wife is also retired.

The second equation (in column 2) indicates considerable similarity to the prediction equation for husbands. Wives who are themselves retired and have husbands who are also retired and satisfied with their activities are more favorable toward retirement. Unlike their husbands, however, income has a slight effect on their retirement attitudes. Specifically, more favorable retirement attitudes are likely among those with lower incomes. Though this relationship is weak, some comment on its unexpected direction is needed. We do not propose that higher income is a detriment to retirement adjustment in general, but rather that wives in households with high incomes are more likely to sense the

Table 6-3
Standardized LISREL Estimates for the Model of Retirement Attitudes of Married Couples
(N = 1,409)

A. *Measurement Model (Factor Loadings)*[a]

Indicators	η_1 Husband, T_1	η_2 Wife, T_1	η_3 Husband, T_2	η_4 Wife, T_2
Y_1	.50			
Y_2	.78			
Y_3	.64			
Y_4		.47		
Y_5		.78		
Y_6		.63		
Y_7			.50	
Y_8			.79	
Y_9			.65	
Y_{10}				.47
Y_{11}				.79
Y_{12}				.63

Total coefficient of determination for Y variables is 0.987.

B. *Structural Equation Model*

Exogenous Variables	η_1	η_2	η_3	η_4
Husband retired[b]	− .33[d]	− .20[e]	− .07[d]	− .04
Activity dissatisfaction	.17[e]	.12[e]		
Household income	.04	.08[d]		
Wife retired[b]	− .13[e]	− .18[e]	− .07[e]	− .12[e]
η_1 (husband, T_1)			.51[e]	.06
η_2 (wife, T_1)			.18[e]	.57[e]

C. *Errors (ω_1) in Equations*[c]

	1	2	3	4
1	.15[e]			
2	.55[e]	.10[e]		
3			.44[e]	
4			.25[e]	.42[e]

Note: χ^2 = 494.1 with 97 degrees of freedom. Goodness of fit index = .747.

[a]All coefficients in the measurement model are significant at $p < .01$. The following measurement errors were found to be significantly correlated: (ϵ_4, ϵ_1), (ϵ_6, ϵ_3), (ϵ_7, ϵ_1), (ϵ_7, ϵ_4), (ϵ_8, ϵ_5), (ϵ_9, ϵ_3), (ϵ_9, ϵ_6), $(\epsilon_{10}, \epsilon_7)$, $(\epsilon_{12}, \epsilon_3)$, $(\epsilon_{12}, \epsilon_6)$, $(\epsilon_{12}, \epsilon_9)$.

[b]Measured in 1977 for the first two equations and 1979 for the last two equations.

[c]Entries on the diagonal are R^2 statistics; off-diagonal entries are correlated errors in equations.

[d]$p < .05$.

[e]$p < .01$.

magnitude of reductions in retirement income and thereby be slightly apprehensive about retirement. As our data suggest in the fourth equation (in column 4), this effect is only temporary as income does not affect change in wives' subsequent retirement attitudes.

Returning to the effects of retirement status on attitudes at time 1 allows us to proffer some conclusions regarding one of our salient research questions. As Atchley [1] stated the question: "How do variations in the retirement status of the husband and wife affect the couple's reaction to retirement?" These results suggest that couples are more favorable toward retirement when both are retired. In addition, the effects of retirement status on retirement attitudes differ for husbands and wives. A husband's attitudes are much more likely to be affected by his retirement than his wife's retirement, whereas a wife's attitudes toward retirement are just about equally influenced by her own retirement and her husband's retirement. (In actuality, his retirement is a slightly stronger predictor of her attitudes than her own retirement).

Turning to the time 2 equations, we can see that there is substantial stability in husbands' retirement attitudes (beta = .51). Changes to increasingly positive attitudes toward retirement are noted for those husbands who are retired and whose wives are also retired. In other words, most married male retirees grow more positive toward retirement, especially when their wives are also retired. Even more important for predicting retired husbands' change in attitudes is their wives' earlier attitudes. If their wives were previously positive, they will become even more positive about retirement. However, if their wives were previously negative, they too will become more negative about retirement.

Wives' changes in attitude is not as substantial as their husbands, as judged by the stability coefficient (beta = .57). What changes do occur are only a function of their own retirement status. Neither their husbands' retirement status nor previous attitudes toward retirement effects any change in their attitudes. This finding lends some support to the research by Kerckhoff [14] which found that wives' attitudes toward retirement are more stable than their husbands. Interestingly, husbands' retirement attitudes are more likely to change and to be influenced by their wives.

Earlier we noted that more favorable attitudes toward retirement are common among couples when both parties are retired. Building upon Lipman's [13] research, we might assert that role convergence produces attitudinal convergence among couples confronting retirement. While there are notable differences in the determinants of retirement attitudes, there is substantial convergence in these attitudes, of a positive tone, especially when role convergence is present. This is also evident in the correlated errors in equations found in section C of table 6-3.

There is moderately strong convergence in retirement attitudes at time 1 net of the exogenous variables ($\psi = .55$). In addition, the change in retirement attitudes of the couples is significantly correlated ($\psi = .25$).

Conclusions

This study has used data gathered in a national sample of older adults to examine the retirement attitudes of married couples. The major findings of our analysis are fivefold. First, older married couples tend to have generally favorable attitudes toward retirement. Second, the most favorable attitudes toward retirement exist among couples who are both retired. Stated more generally, role convergence increases the likelihood of attitudinal convergence. Third, a husband's attitudes toward retirement are much more likely to be affected by his retirement than his wife's retirement, whereas a wife's attitudes toward retirement are just about equally influenced by her own retirement and her husband's retirement. Fourth, while retired couples tend to be stable in their retirement attitudes, wives tend to be somewhat more stable than their husbands. Fifth, change in the retirement attitudes of husbands is more likely to be influenced by their wives than vice versa.

This study, which uses longitudinal data, gives general support to the findings of Kerckhoff [14] based on cross-sectional data. Most notable is confirmation of the finding that wives' retirement attitudes are more stable than their husbands although in our study both husbands and wives showed considerable stability. The changes that do occur among husbands as they retire are substantially affected by their wives. What tends to make them more positive about retirement is not additional income derived from a working spouse, but rather a retired spouse providing consensual validation to the retirement role.

These findings may be generally considered as confirming the continuity theory approach to identity for understanding retirement [4]. Most of these older couples are favorable toward retirement. Even more important, retirement does not create a crisis in attitudinal dispositions for most couples. Retirement attitudes are fairly stable and increasingly positive as both partners become retired.

For those who were more negative about retirement, it was not the act of retiring that developed such attitudes. On the contrary, it was the act of continuing to work that caused some husbands and wives to become more negative about retirement. Also, as one might expect, the decision to continue working is shaped by previous attitudes toward retirement.

Early conceptions of how people experienced life events such as retirement and widowhood were rather simple in terms of how these transitions were believed to affect individuals and families. Increasingly, studies of life events point in the direction of conditional relationships as people face such transitions. This study, by examining the married couple, has specified several conditional relationships for predicting retirement attitudes. Older couples are generally positive about retirement and especially so when both are retired. We can agree with Bernard [16] that there are "his" and "her" marriages, but recognize that the more similarity in the structure of social life the more convergent the marriage.

References

1. R.C. Atchley, "Issues in Retirement Research," *The Gerontologist* 19 (1979):44–54.

2. S.H. Beck, "Adjustment to and Satisfaction with Retirement," *Journal of Gerontology* 37 (1982):616–624.

3. L.K. George and G.L. Maddox, "Subjective Adaptation to Loss of the Work Role: A Longitudinal Study," *Journal of Gerontology* 32 (1977):456–462.

4. E. Mutran and D.C. Reitzes, "Retirement, Identity and Well-Being: Realignment of Role Relationships," *Journal of Gerontology* 36 (1981):733–740.

5. E. Mutran and D.C. Reitzes, "Intergenerational Support Activities and Well-Being," *American Sociological Review* 49 (1984):117–130.

6. R.C. Atchley, *The Sociology of Retirement* (N.Y.: John Wiley & Sons, 1976).

7. E.A. Friedman and H.L. Orbach, "Adjustments to Retirement," in S. Areti (ed.), *American Handbook of Psychiatry* (N.Y.: Basic Books, 1982).

8. G.F. Streib and C.J. Schneider, *Retirement in American Society: Impact and Process* (Ithaca, N.Y.: Cornell University Press, 1971).

9. W.J. Goudy, E.A. Powers, P.M. Keith, and R.A. Reger, "Changes in Attitudes toward Retirement: Evidence from a Panel Study of Older Males," *Journal of Gerontology* 35 (1980):942–948.

10. E.B. Palmore, G.G. Fillenbaum, and L.K. George, "Consequences of Retirement," *Journal of Gerontology* 39 (1984):109–116.

11. J. Tuckman and I. Lorge, *Retirement and the Industrial Worker: Prospect and Reality* (N.Y.: Teachers College Bureau of Publications, 1954).

12. G.F. Streib, "Family Patterns in Retirement," *Journal of Social Issues* 14 (1958):46–60.

13. A. Lipman, "Role Conceptions and Morale of Couples in Retirement," *Journal of Gerontology* 16 (1961):267–271.

14. A.C. Kerckhoff, "Husband-Wife Expectations and Reactions to Retirement," *Journal of Gerontology* 16 (1984):267–271.

15. L.B. Rubin, *Worlds of Pain/Life in the Working Class Family* (N.Y.: Basic Books, 1969).

16. J. Bernard, *The Future of Marriage* (N.Y.: World Publishing Company, 1972).

17. L.M. Irelan, "Retirement History Study: Introduction," *Social Security Bulletin* 35 (1972):24–33.

18. K.G. Joreskog and D. Sorbom, *LISREL V and LISREL VI: Analysis of Linear Structural Relationships by Maximum Likelihood and Least Square Methods* (Chicago: National Education Resources, 1983).

19. B. Wheaton, B. Munthen, D.F. Alwin, and G.F. Summers, "Assessing Reliability and Stability in Panel Models," in D.R. Heise (ed.), *Sociological Methodology* (San Francisco: Jossey-Bass, 1977).

20. D. Sorbom, "Detection of Correlated Errors in Longitudinal Data," *British Journal of Mathematical and Statistical Psychology* 28 (1975):138–151.

21. R.T. Campbell and E. Mutran, "Analyzing Panel Data in Studies of Aging: Applications of the LISREL Model," *Research on Aging* 4 (1982):3–41.

22. K.G. Joreskog, "Structural Analysis of Covariance and Correlation Matrices," *Psychometrika* 43 (1978):443–477.

7

Major Role Losses and Social Participation of Older Males

A recurrent theme in the sociology of aging is that major role losses, such as those experienced in widowhood and retirement, alter social participation with kin and friends and within organizations [1, 2]. While some have suggested that widowhood and retirement actually enhance social participation as individuals attempt to use other groups as functional substitutes for their losses [3, 4], others indicate that these events may result in reduced participation [5]. Among the latter group, one interpretation of these events has been that reduced participation was a result of the role loss itself as a consequence of the individual's desire to disengage from society. Another interpretation, however, might be that major role loss does not in itself reduce social activity. Instead, deteriorative changes associated with the role loss, such as a decline in income or health, may be the important factors contributing to a decline in participation.

An alternative to the proposition that life changes affect participation is that factors which describe a behavioral orientation toward participation developed over the life cycle, what might be called "a participatory life style" [6–8], explain variations in activity in later life. According to this interpretation, personal characteristics such as socioeconomic status, kin network size, and the level of prior participation provide a better clue to understanding the elderly's interaction than changes such as retirement which are experienced toward the end of their lives.

This research investigated the relative salience of major role losses, specifically those experienced in widowhood and retirement, personal characteristics, and prior levels of social participation, to observed variations in informal and formal participation among a group of males in their sixties. In this paper, analytical models were employed to distin-

A reprint from T.T.H. Wan and B.G. Odell, "Major Role Losses and Social Participation of Older Males," *Research On Aging* 5 (1983):173–196. Reprinted by permission of Sage Publications, Inc.

guish sets of variables reflecting changes (widowhood, retirement, and their related deteriorative changes) from other social descriptive variables (kin network size, socioeconomic status, previous participation) in order to determine which factors best facilitate prediction of informal and formal participation. It was hoped that such an examination would suggest whether the direction of future gerontological research and policy in the area of participation should be to continue to explore the impacts of major role losses associated with old age or to vigorously pursue the more complex path of unraveling relevant personal characteristics and patterns developed over the life cycle.

Related Research

It has been argued that loss of the spouse or work role, which is accompanied by a reorganization of remaining roles and often an identity crisis, alters existing patterns of interaction. Following this logic, the study of widowhood and retirement is a prerequisite for our understanding of both informal and formal social participation among the elderly. In fact, Palmore [9], looking at the effects of widowhood and retirement on interpersonal relations, in general found these events increased interpersonal relations. From this he suggests the possibility of substitution for losses experienced. Other literature gives a somewhat different picture of the impact of these events.

Turning specifically to the impact of widowhood on kin relations, it appears that interaction is lower after the death of a spouse [1, 10–12]. There is, however, some contradictory evidence that no differences occur in contact with kin between married and widowed persons [13, 14]. The very few studies that have investigated the consequences of retirement on relations with kin present contradictory conclusions concerning its impact [15].

It appears that friendships in old age may be more vulnerable to the effects of widowhood and retirement than kin relations, as marital and employment status homogeneity have been demonstrated to influence interaction [2]. Although several studies have noted differences between married and widowed and working and retired, whether major role losses increase or decrease participation with friends cannot be decisively ascertained [16, 17]. Although most of the evidence suggests that major role losses experienced in widowhood and retirement influence informal participation, these events do not appear to affect formal participation in organizations [10, 12, 13, 15, 18]. There is only a suggestion that the organizational memberships of retired men decline when the memberships held were associated with the occupational role [19].

Some research has led to speculation that sex could be an intervening variable between major role losses and social participation. Males appear to alter their informal interaction with kin and friends following bereavement while female interaction remains stable [12, 20]. Differences in participation in formal organizations have also been discerned between widowed men and women [1, 21, 22].

It is postulated here that other deteriorative life changes, for example, reduction in health status or income, increases in the propensity to move, and in the course of life dissatisfaction occurring concomitantly with widowhood and retirement, alter participation more than major role losses themselves. It has been demonstrated that these deteriorative change events are associated with widowhood or retirement as well as with low levels of participation [23–27]. The intervening influence of deteriorative changes might help to explain the observed sex differences in adaptation to major role losses as particular changes could occur more often among one sex than another. For example, the findings of Elwell and Maltbie-Crannell [26] indicate that age, income, and health intervene between widowhood and the social participation of males but not females.

To date, consideration of personal characteristics such as socioeconomic status, kin network size, and the previous level of participation as explanatory variables has been obscured by examination of major role losses, even though these foregoing factors have been shown to be relevant to social participation. Socioeconomic status has been positively associated with informal participation with friends and formal participation in organizations [28, 29]. Although kin network size has not been specifically related to the frequency of informal or formal activity, it can be assumed that the availability of kin facilitates informal participation and may contribute to the development of a pattern of interaction over the life cycle. Evidence also indicates that the prior level of interaction determines the need for social activity in old age [30, 31].

Based upon the research literature cited above, it is postulated that major role losses, their related deteriorative changes, personal characteristics, and prior level of interaction all affect participation. Yet questions of their relative importance, their joint effects, and their relevance to specific types of formal and informal interaction remain to be answered in our investigation.

Methodology

Data Source

In our analysis, the effect of widowhood and retirement on social participation was assessed by examining data obtained from the LRHS, which consists of information collected biannually by the Bureau of the Census for the Social Security Administration, in order to study the retirement process. Data were analyzed for the years 1969–1971. A lack of consistency in questions pertaining to social participation, however, required that the dependent variable be examined for a single year 1971, although independent variables were derived longitudinally between 1969/1971, thus utilizing some historical aspects of the data.

From a national sample in 1969 of 11,153 persons between the ages of fifty-eight and sixty-three years, a subsample of 6,603 males was chosen, all of whom were either married or widowed, and working or retired, and had been in either category of both statuses in 1969 and 1971. Females were excluded from this study due to restrictions in the 1969 data which included unmarried females only.

Dependent Variable. Social participation was examined in terms of informal and formal participation. Informal participation was measured by the extent of interaction with children, siblings, parents, spouse's parents, relatives, and friends. For each area of informal participation, frequency of participation in terms of daily, weekly, monthly, and less than monthly was assigned a score of 4, 3, 2, and 1, respectively. Absence of participation was scored as 0. A composite score was based upon the sum of all types of informal participation ranged from 0 to 24.

Formal participation was measured by the number of social and professional organizational memberships held. Correlation analysis of the data showed that formal participation was not significantly related to any specific type of informal interaction or to the composite measure of total informal interaction, a finding which justifies this two-dimensional approach to participation.

Independent Variables. The independent variables included were widowhood and retirement status, amount of related deteriorative life change experienced, socioeconomic status, kin network size, and prior level of social participation.

Widowhood and retirement status were reported by the respondent. Although a more objective method of defining retirement status could have been employed, it was speculated that this self-definition would be indicative of an attitude which would better predict participation.

Deteriorative life change is operationally defined as undesirable changes occurring in the late life. The deteriorative changes experienced by the respondent between 1969 and 1971 included a decline in subjective health status, economic well-being, and life satisfaction; an increase in financial dependence, physical mobility limitation and disability; residential mobility and the departure of children from the household. Financial dependence was defined as being dependent on a sibling or child for regular support. Physical mobility limitation and disability were both assessed by measures marking increased levels of limitation. For instance, mobility limitation was defined incrementally as needing transportation, being housebound, and being bedridden. While it might have been anticipated that some of the eight deteriorative life changes examined would be associated, correlation analysis proved this not to be the case. We found that there were no significant correlations among these deteriorative change events.

Socioeconomic status comprised a three-factor index of income, education, and occupation. Based upon the procedure suggested by Green [32], each factor was differentially weighted on the basis of race, white or nonwhite.

Kin network consisted of the presence of living children, parents, siblings, spouse's parents, and spouse's siblings reported by the respondent. A total score was computed, ranging from 0 to 57.

Previous participation was assessed for informal and formal participation. Previous informal participation was based on a summary measure of frequency of interaction with several types of kin (parents, spouse's parents, children, and siblings) in 1969. Previous formal participation was based on the number of social or professional memberships held in 1969.

Analytic Approach

The analysis presented here is in two parts. In the first part, step-wise regression analysis was employed to assess the importance of combinations of independent variables as well as the effect of single variables in accounting for the variance in social participation. Four separate regression analyses were performed. Model I included widowhood and retirement status as predictor variables. Model II added another variable, amount of deteriorative life change experienced, to model I. Model III included socioeconomic status, kin network size, and prior level of informal and formal participation alone. Model IV was a summary model including all of the six predictor variables. Examination of the beta coefficient for each predictor in these models reveals the relative contribution of each variable in explaining the variance in the dependent variable after controlling for other predictors.

In the second part of the analysis, Multiple Classification Analysis was used to further explore two other pertinent questions: (1) What is the effect of a major role loss on the mean level of participation after adjusting for other relevant variables?, and (2) What is the effect of recency of a major role loss on the mean level of participation? Multiple

Classification Analysis is a technique which examines the gross effect of a predictor when taken by itself as well as its net effect after adjustments are made for intercorrelations with other predictors [33]. This technique differs from regression in that, in this analysis, differences within categories of a predictor can be observed. The effects of widowhood and retirement on mean informal and formal participation was examined separately after controlling for socioeconomic status, kin network size, prior level of participation, deteriorative life change, and experiencing another major role loss (either widowhood or retirement). Categories of marital and retirement status were subdivided by whether the status change occurred prior to 1969 or between 1969–1971 in order to determine the effect of recency of the role loss. Thus, four groups formed on the basis of marital status were (1) married 1969/married 1971; (2) married 1969/widowed 1971; (3) widowed 1969/married 1971; and (4) widowed 1969/widowed 1971. Corresponding groups were formed on the basis of the retirement status.

Results

Table 7–1 displays the distribution of selected characteristics for the entire study sample by widowhood and by retirement status. The sample which was 9% widowed and 39% retired had a mean age of 62.39 years, mean socioeconomic status of 56.97, and mean kin network size of 9.28 persons in 1971. As a whole, the sample experienced very few deteriorative life changes in the areas specified.

Comparing married with widowed males, we found there were significant differences in age, socioeconomic status, kin network size, and the total amount of deteriorative life change experienced. Widowed males were slightly older, had lower socioeconomic status, and smaller kin networks than the married. They were more likely to be retired. Widowed males also experienced a greater mean number of deteriorative changes (1.32) than the married (.98), and a greater percentage of widowed (15.2%) than married (7.4%) had at least three or more deteriorative changes during the two-year period studied.

Significant differences between retired and nonretired males appeared in age, socioeconomic status, widowed status, and the amount of deteriorative life change experienced. The retired were on the average older and more likely to be widowed. Being retired, however, was not related to lower socioeconomic status as was being widowed. In fact, retirees had a higher socioeconomic status score than nonretirees. The retired also had a greater mean number of deteriorative changes (1.15) compared to the nonretired (.91) and a greater percentage had three or more deteriorative changes (11.39% compared to 6.1%).

Table 7-1
Selected Characteristics of the Study Sample in 1971 by Widowhood and Retirement Status
(N = 6,603)

	Number	Mean Age	Mean SES Score	Mean Kin Network Size	% Widowed	% Retired	Mean LCE Indicating Decline	% with Three or More LCE Indicating Decline
Total	6,603	62.39	56.97	9.28	8.8	39.1	1.01	8.2
Widowhood status								
Widowed	581	62.63	55.16	6.16	8.89	50.5	1.32	15.2
Married	6,022	62,36	57.14	9.58	91.27	38.0	0.98	7.4
Significant differences between the widowed and the married		0.27[a]	−2.02[a]	−3.42[a]	82.31[a]	11.5[a]	0.34[a]	7.8[a]
Retirement status								
Retired	2,586	63.12	59.59	9.30	11.2	39.1	1.15	11.3
Nonretired	4,017	61.91	55.15	9.27	7.0	60.9	0.91	6.1
Significant differences between the retired and the nonretired		1.21[a]	4.64[a]	0.03	4.2[a]	21.8[a]	0.24[a]	5.2[a]

Note: SES = Socioeconomic status.
LCE = Deteriorative life change events.
[a] $p < .01$.

The fact that a higher mean number of deteriorative life changes, as well as a larger percentage of respondents experiencing three or more deteriorative changes, was found among both the widowed and retired implies that the occurrence of deteriorative change in the areas specified may be concomitant with major role losses. Correlation analysis shows, however, that specific deteriorative changes are not significantly associated with either widowhood or retirement status, nor are they correlated with specific types of informal or formal participation. Correlation analysis does reveal that it is not specific deterioration changes, but rather experiencing the cumulative effects of several deteriorative changes which distinguishes the widowed and retired from their counterparts.

The first stage of our analysis, as shown in tables 7-2 and 7-3, discerned the relative contribution of widowhood, retirement, and the other independent variables—deteriorative life change, socioeconomic status, kin network size, and previous participation—in explaining variance in the dependent variable, social participation, when these variables were viewed as combined entities and as single predictors.

From a first glance at table 7-2, it is apparent that all four proposed models explain more variance in formal (at the maximum level of 31.1%) than in informal participation (maximum 6.2% participation with parents), suggesting that the variables studied are better predictors of participation in formal organizations.

As could have been anticipated, model IV, which comprised all of the above predictors, explained the largest amount of variance in informal and formal participation. It is interesting to note that differences between model IV and model III, including personal characteristics and prior level of participation, are not great, while differences between model III and model II, comprising widowhood, retirement, and amount of deteriorative change experienced, are. While model III accounts for almost 3% of the variance in total informal participation, model II accounts for only 0.3%. In formal participation, model III accounts for almost 29% of the variance, and model II explains only about 2%, revealing a difference of 27% between two models.

The difference in total explained variance between models I and II is negligible, indicating that the inclusion of related deteriorative change in the model II does not enhance our understanding of social participation. It appears that experiencing deteriorative change, such as increasing disability, or a decline in health or income, did not substantially affect formal and informal activity of men in this age group.

Table 7-3 indicates the net effect (beta) of each variable within a specific model while simultaneously controlling for the effects of other variables. Examination of model IV, which included all of the indepen-

Table 7-2
Proportions of Variance in Informal and Formal Social Participation Explained by Major Role Losses, Concomitant Life Changes, Personal Characteristics, and Previous Social Participation

		Informal Participation						Formal Participation
Predictors	Total	SP1	SP2	SP3	SP4	SP5	SP6	
Major role losses alone	0.3[a]	0.2[a]	0.2[a]	0.1	2.2[a]	0.3[a]	0.2[a]	2.0[a]
Major role losses plus concomitant life changes	0.3[a]	0.2[b]	0.2[b]	0.2[b]	2.2[a]	0.3[a]	0.2	2.2[a]
Personal characteristics and previous social participation	2.9[a]	2.9[a]	2.2[a]	0.2[b]	3.5[a]	5.6[a]	0.2	28.8[a]
All factors combined: (2) + (3)	3.2[a]	3.3[a]	2.3[a]	0.4[b]	5.0[a]	6.2[a]	0.6[b]	31.1[a]

Note: SP = overall informal social participation
SP1 = with children
SP2 = with siblings
SP3 = with relatives
SP4 = with spouse's parents
SP5 = with parents
SP6 = with friends

[a] $p < .001$.
[b] $p < .05$.

Table 7–3
Summary Statistics from Regression Analysis of Social Participation by Selected Predictors

	Informal Participation							
	Model 1		Model 2		Model 3		Model 4	
	B	Beta	B	Beta	B	Beta	B	Beta
Predictors								
Widowhood	−.258	−.023	−.246	−.022			−.163	−.014
Retirement	−.309[b]	−.048	−.301[b]	−.047			−.309[b]	−.048
Deteriorative life change			−.036	−.011			−.034	−.011
SES					.005	.019	.009[a]	.028
Kin network size					−.015	−0.24	−0.15	−.024
Previous participation								
Informal					.239[b]	.173	.236[b]	.171
Formal							.002	.002
Mean	9.56		9.56		9.31		9.29	
R^2	0.003		0.003		0.028		0.031	

	Formal Participation							
	Model 1		Model 2		Model 3		Model 4	
	B	Beta	B	Beta	B	Beta	B	Beta
Predictors								
Widowhood	−.680[b]	−.088	−.650[b]	−.084			−.464[b]	−.060
Retirement	−.484[b]	−.108	−.463[b]	−.103			−.584[b]	−.130
Deteriorative life change			−.092[b]	−.042			−.060[a]	−.027
SES					.045[b]	.205	.051[b]	.236
Kin network size					−.023[b]	−.051	−.028[b]	−.063
Previous participation								
Informal					.020[a]	.021		
Formal					.299[b]	.439	.284[b]	.418
Mean	4.65		4.64		3.38		3.27	
R^2	0.020		0.022		0.288		0.311	

Note: Model 1 refers to an analysis of the effect of retirement and widowhood on social participation.

Model 2 includes retirement, widowhood, and deteriorative life change events as predictors.

Model 3 includes SES, kin network size, and previous participation as predictors.

Model 4 includes all six factors combined.

[a]$p < .05$.

[b]$p < .01$.

dent variables under study, shows that three significant predictors of total informal activity, in descending order of importance, are (1) prior level of informal participation (beta = .171); (2) retirement status (beta = .048); and (3) socioeconomic status (beta = .028). While prior level of participation and socioeconomic status are positively associated with participation, retirement is negatively related. It is noteworthy that in model IV, previous levels of informal activity are by far the best predictors of current informal activity.

Turning to informal participation, examination of model IV shows that the effects of all of the independent variables considered are statistically significant. Their order of importance is ranked as follows: (1) prior level of formal participation (beta = .418); (2) socioeconomic status (beta = .236); (3) retirement status (beta = .130); (4) kin network size (beta = .063); (5) widowhood status (beta = .060); (6) deteriorative life change (beta = .027); and (7) prior level of informal participation (beta = 0.21). As was found with informal activity, prior levels of participation (in this case the prior level of formal activity) were the best predictors of current formal participation. The higher the level of previous formal and informal activity in 1969, and the higher the level of socioeconomic status in 1971, the greater the participation in formal organizations.

In analyzing the four models, we found that widowhood and related deteriorative change factors are less important than prior level of activity and socioeconomic status in explaining participation. Retirement is less important than prior level of activity to informal and formal participation and less relevant than socioeconomic status to formal participation.

In the second stage, Multiple Classification Analysis was performed to look at the effects of widowhood and retirement on mean levels of participation, after adjusting for other variables. The results shown in tables 7–4 and 7–5 indicate significant differences between the married and widowed, and the retired and nonretired in several areas. In general, both major role losses appear to reduce participation in formal organizations and tend to be associated with lower levels of informal interaction. Table 7–4 indicates significant differences in participation on the basis of marital status in the area of total informal participation and interaction with children, parents, spouse's parents, friends, and in formal participation defined by the number of memberships held in professional and social organizations. No significant differences occurred in participation with siblings or other relatives.

Results indicate that those recently remarried (widowed 1969/married 1971) were the highest participators in the areas of total informal participation, participation with spouse's parents, friends, and in orga-

Table 7-4
Adjusted Means of Social Participation by Marital Status (1969 and 1971) and Types of Social Participation in 1971

Marital Status	Types of Social Participation							
	Total Informal	Children	Siblings	Relatives	Parents	Spouse's Parents	Friends	Formal Organization
Married (1969 & 1971) (N = 5,990)	4.15	1.19	0.67	0.69	0.31	0.57	0.70	1.35
Widowed (1969)/married (1971) (N = 32)	5.42	0.97	1.04	0.72	0.28	1.41	1.02	1.68
Married (1969)/widowed (1971) (N = 335)	4.21	1.12	0.70	0.79	0.56	0.10	0.92	0.75
Widowed (1969 & 1971) (N = 246)	3.69	0.93	0.70	0.77	0.32	0.19	0.78	0.98
F-value	4.46[b]	3.78[b]	1.59	1.08	9.93[b]	28.82[b]	3.27[a]	21.31[b]

Note: Adjusted mean of social participation was obtained from Multiple Classification Analysis in which the effects of retirement status in both 1969 and 1971, deteriorative life change events, SES, kin network size, and previous levels of social participation were simultaneously controlled.

[a]$p < 0.05$.
[b]$p < 0.01$.

Table 7-5
Adjusted Means of Social Participation by Retirement Status (1969 and 1971) and Types of Social Participation in 1971

Retirement Status	Types of Social Participation							
	Total Informal	Children	Siblings	Relatives	Parents	Spouse's Parents	Friends	Formal Organization
Not retired (1969 & 1971) (N = 3,853)	4.27	1.24	0.67	0.72	0.36	0.57	0.69	1.50
Retired (1969)/not retired (1971) (N = 164)	4.13	1.19	0.54	0.65	0.35	0.78	0.61	1.41
Not retired (1969)/retired (1971) (N = 1,348)	3.96	1.12	0.65	0.66	0.29	0.45	0.79	1.04
Retired (1969 & 1971) (N = 1,238)	3.94	1.07	0.70	0.68	0.21	0.52	0.75	0.99
F-value	7.23[a]	6.33[a]	1.49	1.62	11.44[a]	5.91[a]	2.27	64.24[a]

Note: Adjusted mean of social participation was obtained from Multiple Classification Analysis in which the effects of marital status in both 1969 and 1971, deteriorative life change events, SES, kin network size, and previous levels of social participation were simultaneously controlled.

[a] $p < 0.01$.

nizations. They also had the highest degree of participation with sib-lings, although this area was not significant. Those married two or more years (married 1969/married 1971) also exhibited high levels of partici-pation with children, spouse's parents, and in organizations.

The widowed show a higher degree of participation than the married in only a few selected areas, and there is great variation in participation among the widowed depending upon the length of the widowed period. Those recently bereaved (married 1969/widowed 1971) had the highest level of participation with parents and the second highest degree of par-ticipation with children and friends among the four groups studied. Those widowed two years or more did not have high levels of participa-tion in any area and showed the lowest level of total informal participa-tion with children.

The recency of the major role loss, termed the recency effect, is a crucial consideration in interpreting these results. Recent remarriage seems to stimulate these men's interaction outside the nuclear family with their new spouse's parents, friends, and in the holding of organiza-tional memberships. These men may also pick up interaction with chil-dren after the low levels experienced in widowhood. In any case, there is a clear pattern of branching out in this group which contrasts with the pattern of the recently bereaved, which is characterized by dropping out of formal activity and drawing upon kin for support as exhibited by high levels of interaction with parents and children and even with other rela-tives, although this latter area is not significant. It is interesting to note that interaction with friends is highest among the recently remarried and recently bereaved, inferring that in times of change, friends may be a source of support against stress.

Table 7–5 reveals significant differences among the four categories of retired and nonretired studied in total informal participation and interaction with children, parents, spouse's parents, and in formal orga-nizations. Differences were not significant in interaction with siblings, other relatives, or friends.

Unlike the widowed where the greatest extremes in social participa-tion scores occurred between those who were recently bereaved or recently married, the greatest extremes between those retired and non-retired occurred among those who had a particular status for two or more years. Men reported nonretired in 1969 and 1971, whom we assume were consistently working during this period, had the highest levels of total informal participation, interaction with children and par-ents, and the greatest number of memberships in formal organizations. These men also maintained relatively high levels of interaction with spouse's parents, siblings, and other relatives, although differences in these two latter areas were not significant. On the other hand, men retired for two or more years had the lowest levels of total informal as well as formal participation. They also revealed a low interaction with spouse's parents.

The fact that retirement does not significantly affect interaction with siblings, other relatives, and friends implies that this event is not detrimental to participation with age peers for whom the respondent has no responsibility.

The negative effects of widowhood and retirement on social participation that were found even when controlling for personal characteristics, prior level of participation, and related deteriorative change are exacerbated when the cumulative effects of experiencing both major role losses are examined. Examination of data for both 1969 and 1971 shows that men who are both widowed and retired have a lower level of total informal and formal participation than men with one or no role losses. Conversely, those who have no role losses have the highest level of participation.

Moreover, the influence of the recency effect, noted when the influence of widowhood and retirement were considered individually, is more evident in formal participation when the cumulative effects of these events are considered. While the ratio of married/working men's formal memberships to those of the widowed/retired was 1.6 to 1 in 1969, this ratio increased to 3 to 1 in 1971 with the inclusion of those who recently changed marital or retirement status or both. Joint consideration of widowhood and retirement did not substantially increase the recency effect in informal participation.

Conclusions

Our findings suggest that the participatory life style developed in the preretirement stage has more influence on social participation than major role losses and other deteriorative changes experienced in old age. Continuity factors which depict this participatory life style, such as socioeconomic status, kin network size, and prior level of activity are better predictors of participation than factors which reflect the experience of change such as widowhood and retirement.

It is interesting to note that the effect of role losses such as widowhood and retirement on social participation was stronger than that of the concomitant declines in subjectively assessed health, income, and life satisfaction, the increases in disability, financial dependence, and limitations on physical mobility, and the departure of children from the family. This leads us to infer that complex psychological factors incumbent upon major role losses may affect participation more substantially than specific deprivations such as income loss.

Looking at the effects of the predictors on social participation, the level of participation two years prior to this study was the single most important predictor of current informal and formal participation. Socioeconomic status and retirement status were also strong predictors of informal and formal participation although they accounted for considerably more variance in formal than in informal participation. While prior level of activity and socioeconomic status were both positively related to social participation, being retired was related to a decline in activity. The inclusion of retirement but not widowhood among the most important predictors encourages us to speculate that for men, at least, loss of the work role has more extensive effects than loss of spouse.

The findings concerning the individual and combined effects of these variables imply that a model consisting of prior level of activity and personal characteristics provides a better basis for understanding interaction with kin and friends and membership in organizations than a model focusing on major role losses alone or role losses in combination with other deteriorative changes. However, it should not be concluded that either role losses or prior participatory behavior and personal characteristics should be employed exclusively. The combined effect of all independent variables considered in this study explained over 30% of the variance in organizational membership, providing a good model for understanding formal activity. On the other hand, findings that the foregoing account for only 3% of the variance in total informal interaction imply that variables not included in this study, for example, the proximity of kin, the quality of the interaction, and the attitude toward specific types of participation, may be more predictive of informal participation.

Certainly, given the importance of prior level of activity and socioeconomic status, it is necessary to control for these factors in future research when assessing the effect of widowhood and retirement on activity with kin, friends, and in organizations. When the effects of prior activity, socioeconomic status, kin network size, the amount of deteriorative life change, and additional major role loss experienced were simultaneously controlled, we were able to detect a so-called recency effect, defined as the varying influence on an event depending upon whether it occurred prior to 1969 or between 1969–1971. Referring to widowhood status, findings showed men recently remarried (widowed 1969/married 1971) and recently bereaved (married 1969/widowed 1971) had more diverse participation patterns than those who experienced status changes before 1969. As noted, these findings may indicate a branching out of the newly remarried and a narrowing of interests by the widowed. The latter finding lends support to the idea that major role losses themselves lead to withdrawal from kin, friends, and organizations. It may be, however, that withdrawal occurs only from less meaningful relationships, while substitution for spouse may occur in other areas. For instance, higher rates of interaction with parents suggest that an elderly mother, the most likely parental survivor of an elderly widower, may for a time replace his spouse.

Contrary to the effects of marital status when the effects of retirement status were examined, differences in social participation were more exaggerated as the length of the working or retirement period increased, implying a more long-term influence of this variable. It appears that even though the decline in activity was more gradual following retirement than it was after bereavement, withdrawal from formal and selected informal activity does occur. It should be observed, however, that retirement status did not affect interaction with siblings, relatives, or friends, leading to speculation that this event has less impact on association with age peers than on interaction with other generations.

Overall our findings tend to corroborate those of the previous research in the area of informal interaction [1, 12, 16, 17, 34]. Evidence showing that widowhood and retirement are associated with a decline in formal participation, however, is in contradiction to past research which has found that these events have no effect on formal participation [12, 13]. Several explanations for this contradiction are in order. First, this study excluded females while most previous research included both sexes. It may be that the female pattern of formal participation differs from males. Second, participation in this study was assessed by number of memberships held while other studies measure the frequency of activity. Differences found on the basis of retirement status may be accounted for by job-related memberships held by the nonretired.

In view of the above discussions, several recommendations for social policy and research on aging can be made. In the area of policy, preretirement education should encourage social participation at all stages in the life cycle and make men aware of the function of kin networks, friendships, and organizational memberships as sources of support in times of crisis. Given the importance of prior level of participation in predicting current participation, particularly formal activity, it is clear that the ability to rely upon persons or groups as resources must be cultivated earlier in life. Further, organizations should make special efforts to maintain involvement of men who become retired or widowed. Perhaps a buddy system for attending meetings, using persons with similar losses, might overcome fears of no longer being part of the group. Having discerned through this endeavor factors affecting the level and patterns of social participation, future research may clarify ways in which participation serves as a support mechanism to alleviate stress associated with change in later life.

In this chapter, the relationship of widowhood, retirement, personal characteristics, and prior level of activity to the social participation of the elderly was ascertained. Our findings are summarized by the following: (1) when the effects of prior participation, kin network size, and socioeconomic status were considered, these variables explained far more variance in informal and formal participation than either major role losses alone or major role losses plus the amount of concomitant, deteriorative life change experienced; (2) the combined effects of socioeconomic status, kin network size, and prior level of participation accounted for more variance in formal than informal participation; (3) although the widowed and retired experience more deteriorative life changes than their counterparts, consideration of the amount of deteriorative change experienced in addition to the effect of major role losses did not increase explained variance in the dependent variable.

Having determined the relative importance of the foregoing variables, a second analysis was performed to examine the effect of widowhood and retirement on participation while other factors (for example, socioeconomic status, kin network size, prior level of participation, extent of deteriorative life change, and extent of major role loss experienced) were simultaneously controlled. Results indicated that (1) major role loss was associated with lower levels of several types of informal interaction and (2) the cumulative effects of experiencing both major role losses produced a synergistic effect on informal and formal participation. This latter finding leads up to conclude that being married eases adjustment to retirement and working eases adjustment to widowhood.

It is suggested that the above findings have policy implications for preretirement education to point out the relevance of social relationships as support mechanisms in crisis and for developing outreach programs to sustain memberships in formal organizations.

References

1. F.M. Berardo, "Widowhood Status in the United States: Perspective on a Neglected Aspect of the Family Life Cycle," *The Family Coordinator* 17 (1968):191–203.

2. Z. Blau, "Structural Constraints on Friendship in Old Age," *American Sociological Review* 26 (1961):429–439.

3. I. Rosow, *Social Integration of the Aged* (N.Y.: Free Press, 1967).

4. B.D. Bell, "The Family Life Cycle: Primary Relationships and Social Participation Patterns," *The Gerontologist* 13 (1973):78–81.

5. E. Cummings and W. Henry, *Growing Old: The Process of Disengagement* (N.Y.: Basic Books, 1961).

6. R.C. Atchley, "Retirement and Leisure Participation: Continuity or Crisis," *The Gerontologist* 11 (1971):13–17.

7. B. Neugarten and R. Havinghurst, "Personality and Patterns of Aging," in B. Neugarten (ed.), *Middle Age and Aging* (Chicago: University of Chicago Press, 1972).

8. B. Neugarten, "Aging in the Year 2000: The Future of the Young-Old," *The Gerontologist* 15 (1975):4–9.

9. E.B. Palmore, "Predictors of Successful Aging," *The Gerontologist* 19 (1979):427–431.

10. R. Videback and A. Knox, "Alternative Participatory Responses to Aging," in A.M. Rose and W. Peterson (eds.), *Older People and Their Social World* (Philadelphia: F.A. Davis Company, 1965).

11. H.Z. Lopata, "The Social Involvement of American Widows," *American Behavioral Scientist* 14 (1970):41–57.

12. C.T. Pihlblad and D.L. Adams, "Widowhood, Social Participation, and Life Satisfaction," *Aging and Human Development* 3 (1972):323–330.

13. M. Petrowsky, "Marital Status, Sex, and the Social Networks of the Elderly," *Journal of Marriage and the Family* 38 (1976):749–756.

14. G. Rosenberg, *The Worker Grows Old* (San Francisco: Jossey-Bass, 1970).

15. G.F. Streib, "Intergenerational Relations: Perspectives on Two Generations of the Older Parent," *Journal of Marriage and the Family* 27 (1965): 469–476.

16. M. Zborowski and L.D. Eyde, "Aging and Social Participation," *Journal of Gerontology* 17 (1962):424–430.

17. E.A. Powers and G.L. Bultena, "Sex Differences in Intimate Friendships of Old Age," *Journal of Marriage and the Family* 38 (1976):739–747.

18. C. Harvey and H. Bahr, "Widowhood, Morale, and Affiliation," *Journal of Marriage and the Family* 36 (1974):97–106.

19. H.A. Rosencranz, C.T. Pihlblad, and T.E. McNevin, *Social Participation of Older People in a Small Town* (Columbia: Department of Sociology, University of Missouri, 1968).

20. L. Robins and M. Tomanec, "Closeness to Blood Relatives Outside the Immediate Family," *Marriage and Family Living* 24 (1962):340–346.

21. R.C. Atchley, "Dimensions of Widowhood in Later Life," *The Gerontologist* 15 (1975):175–178.

22. K.F. Ferraro and C.M. Barresi, "The Impact of Widowhood on the Social Relations of Older Persons," *Research on Aging* 4 (1982):227–248.

23. D. Maddison and A. Viola, "The Health of Widows in the Year Following Bereavement," *Journal of Psychosomatic Research* 12 (1968):297–306.

24. W. Rees and S. Lutkins, "Mortality of Bereavement," *British Medical Journal* 5 (1967):13–16.

25. H.Z. Lopata, "Widows as a Minority Group," *The Gerontologist* 11 (1971):67–77.

26. F. Elwell and A.D. Maltbie-Crannell, "The Impact and Interaction Effects on Widowhood: Two Models of Empirical Test." Paper presented at the 31st Annual Meeting of the Gerontological Society, Dallas, 1978.

27. G.B. Thompson, "Work Versus Leisure Roles: An Investigation of Morale among Employed and Retired Men," *Journal of Gerontology* 28 (1973): 339–344.

28. N. Babchuck and A. Booth, "Voluntary Association Membership: A Longitudinal Analysis," *American Sociological Review* 34 (1969):31–35.

29. S.J. Cutler, "Aging and Voluntary Association Participation," *Journal of Gerontology* 32 (1976):470–479.

30. M.F. Lowenthal, "Social Isolation and Mental Illness in Old Age," *American Sociological Review* 29 (1964):119–132.

31. P. Townsend and S. Tunstall, "Isolation, Desolation and Loneliness," in E. Shanas (ed.), *Older People in Three Industrial Societies* (N.Y.: Anontherton Press 1968).

32. L.W. Green, "Manual for Scoring Socioeconomic Status for Research on Health Behavior," *Public Health Reports* 85 (1970):815–827.

33. F. Andrews, J.A. Morgan, and J.N. Sonquist, *Multiple Classification Analysis* (Ann Arbor: Institute for Social Research, University of Michigan, 1969).

34. F.M. Berardo, "Survivorship and Social Isolation: The Case of the Aged Widower," *The Family Coordinator* 19 (1970):11–25.

8
Planning for Health and Social Well-Being of the Elderly: A Targeting Approach

A number of social issues are emerging as major forces to shape public policy on aging. These include the growth of the aged population and their demand for care, the decrease of resources being earmarked for support services due to budget constraints, and the continual tightening of the Medicare/Medicaid reimbursement system which affects the delivery of geriatric services in the community. In light of these environmental perplexities, the need for making efficient use of diminishing resources is imperative. A method for targeting the elderly population for services has yet to be developed. For example, identification of elderly persons who have concomitantly experienced ill health, functional incapacities, and life dissatisfaction in the later years may indicate needs for health and social interventions.

The purpose of this chapter is to provide social and health profiles of the frail elderly and identify the characteristics of those who have been adversely affected by role losses such as retirement and widowhood. This identification will facilitate targeting the elderly for improving their access to care. By providing a methodology whereby subpopulations are clustered by the level of frailty, the most needy can be identified so that services may then be specifically channeled to those groups. This type of targeting allocation scheme is essential for the provision of appropriate services to the needy.

Related Research

Recent studies have examined the factors that affect the use of health and social services among the elderly [1–4]. While there are a number of variables (need factors, enabling factors, and predisposing factors) cited as important determinants of utilization, health status, an indicator of the need for care, has been found to be one of the most important predictors of health services use among the elderly [5–7]. Yet no consistent agreement has been made in regard to the measure of need for care. This dilemma may be derived from conceptual and measurement problems of health status. If one utilizes an all-encompassing definition of health status such as "a state of complete physical, mental, and social well-being" as offered by the World Health Organization, one can readily see the problem in quantifying such a diffuse definition of health. Furthermore, if one uses an all-encompassing view of health, a majority of elders could be defined as in a state of poor health and, subsequently, in need of care.

Previous research has included both subjective (self-assessed) and objective (professionally evaluated) measures of health status as indicators of need for services. The presence of chronic conditions, however, does not necessarily reflect the extent of the functional disability of an elderly person. Similarly, self-perceived health status may not fully indicate the level of services needed. Since many elders are afflicted with chronic conditions which may or may not limit their ability to engage in activities of daily living, a further specification of levels of service needs for the frail elderly is urgently needed. This approach should not only identify the functionally disabled elderly in terms of self-assessment and professional assessment, but also match their needs with specific social and health services. Questions which need to be addressed include: Can health and social well-being determine the level of need for health services? What are the major characteristics of those who have shown the need for care but use very few health services? Do high users of physician services actually show more severe need for care than nonusers? What are the determinants of older adults' utilization behavior in later life?

In defining the level of use, there are a number of ways in which normative standards can be produced. For instance, a nominal group approach using a panel of experts, such as the severity index developed for Diagnostic Related Groupings [8], would be one of the methods to create norms of health services use. Statistical norms based upon the mean or median would be another. One study employed the latter to discern high (above average), medium (average), and low (lower than average) users of health services [6]. The ability to define norms for functionally disabled elders will aid the targeting of resources and services to subgroups that are most in need of them. Limited research on targeting resources has been done in the past [9, 10]. Recently, there is a national interest in developing channeling programs such as Triage (Connecticut), Access (Genesee, New York), and Robert Wood Johnson Foundation Project in coordinating comprehensive care for the chronically impaired elderly. While these demonstration projects have examined targeting methodologies in earnest, there have been problems with their methodological framework. These demonstration projects have primarily dealt with major demographic and social characteristics as well as a selection of specific health attributes which best characterize the study groups. Whether it is possible to identify the subpopulations for whom intervention will lead to better patient outcomes or to a reduction in the cost of care is a critical research questions that needs to be built into its evaluation scheme.

In summary, appropriate identification of frail elders through targeting methodologies will enable gerontological specialists, policy makers, and planners to direct services to the most needy.

Methodology

The primary source of data is based upon the LRHS. A selected panel sample of 2,293 older adults who had completed information was used for the present analysis.

Several indexes were constructed and used as the dependent variables. For example, a composite index of physical health—measured by three dummy variables of perceived poor health, disability, and mobility limitation—was computed by summing the values of three health indicators for each of the last three waves of LRHS data (1975, 1977, and 1979). Similarly, an index of social well-being was computed from three dummy social well-being indicators, namely unhappy feelings, life dissatisfaction, and poor economic well-being status. The scores of each of the composite indexes ranged from 0 (the best) to 3 (the poorest) on the physical or social well-being level. The social, demographic, economic, and initial health characteristics of those who had experienced a poor level of physical health or social well-being in 1977 were independently portrayed from a multivariate approach. Furthermore, those who had the poorest level of both physical health and social well-being were identified as the frail elderly by using the same analytic procedures.

In this chapter, we performed statistical analyses of LRHS data in terms of two steps. First, the Automatic Interaction Detector (AID) analysis was used to identify initial (1975) health and social profiles of the elderly who had experienced poor physical health or negative social well-being in 1977. The AID technique is based on one-way analysis of variance and employs a nonsymmetrical branching technique in which the sample is subdivided into a series of mutually exclusive subgroups. This technique is especially suitable for the purpose of clustering the study sample into several subgroups so that individuals within the same group may have similar levels of health and social service needs, while the between-group differences in the need for care may be maximized.

By identifying homogenous subgroups, one can then target the selected individuals for services or interventions. The usefulness and appropriateness of AID in a large-scale survey study has been detailed by Sonquist, Baker, and Morgan [11]; Andersen, Smedby, and Anderson [12]; and Wan and Livieratos [13].

In the second step of analysis, we used Multiple Classification Analysis, which provides information about the relative contribution of each predictor variable to variation in the dependent variable "physician contacts" or "total family income" measured in the last wave of LRHS. This technique shows the effect of each independent variable with and without adjustment for other variables. This analysis will point out the social differentials in health services use and in income of the elderly. It also provides proof of the validity of the frailty classification developed in the first-stage analysis, if the classification can differentiate the utilization and income level of the study population.

Results

Social and Health Profiles of Persons Experiencing Poor Health in Later Life

Figure 8-1 shows the predictor trees for the AID analysis of the physical health index (1977) by selected sociodemographic variables and two lagged well-being variables (prior levels of physical health and social well-being). The prior health level proves to be the most important predictor variable in the AID analysis since it contributes the largest proportion of total variance in health status (table 8-1) and makes a dichotomized split of the total group into two subgroups. The second important variable "dissatisfaction with current activities" makes the further split of the two parent groups (groups 2 and 3) into six final subgroups (groups 6, 7, 8, 9, 10, and 11). It is interesting to note that individuals who experienced the worst health status in 1977 were those (group 11) who had poor health in 1975 and were also dissatisfied with their current activities (mean health index $\bar{Y}$ = 2.3). Other sociodemographic variables, however, did not account for much of the total variation in health status in 1977. This implies that no distinct social profiles of physical health can be ascertained by identifying their social and demographic characteristics.

A similar AID analysis of the health status index in 1979 was performed. The results consistently pointed out that the prior level of health status (1977) was the most important predictor variable of health status in 1979 (table 8-2). Figure 8-2 reveals the predictor trees for the

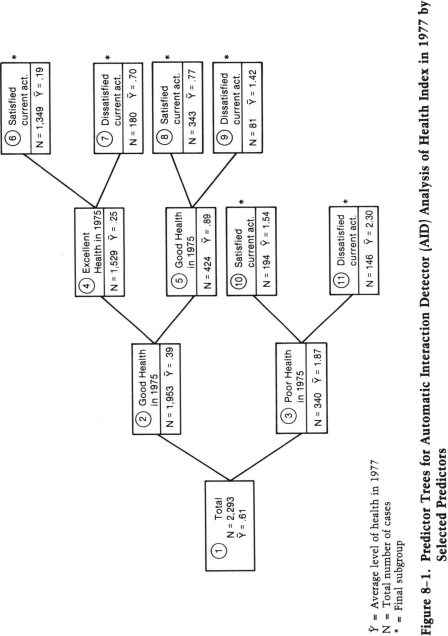

Ȳ = Average level of health in 1977
N = Total number of cases
* = Final subgroup

Figure 8–1. Predictor Trees for Automatic Interaction Detector (AID) Analysis of Health Index in 1977 by Selected Predictors

Table 8–1
Automatic Interaction Detector Analysis of the Relative Contribution of Selected Sociodemographic Variables and Lagged Health and Social Well-Being (SWB) Variables in Explaining Variance in Physical Health (N = 2,293)

	Physical Health Index[a]	
	1977	1979
Predictors		
Lagged health variable	33.49	39.41
Lagged SWB variable	3.75	8.79
Age	0.16	0.10
Sex	1.24	2.36
Race	0.77	0.62
Recency of retirement	2.75	1.48
Recency of widowhood	2.02	5.26
Income levels	2.94	3.65
Participation in senior center activities	0.59	0.84
Dissatisfaction with present activities	17.10	10.13
Number of living children	1.67	1.66
R^2 (% variation explained)	46.90	49.70

[a]A composite index ranging from 0 (excellent health) to 3 (poor health) was computed.

AID analysis of the health index in 1979. Five final groups (groups 2, 8, 9, 6, and 7) emerged from the split of the parent group. Again, we found that individuals who had the poorest level of physical health in 1979 were those who had very poor health in 1977 ($\bar{Y} = 2.37$). Relatively speaking, the recent widows or widowers (group 9) also experienced poorer health status ($\bar{Y} = 1.89$).

Based upon the above findings, we can portray the major characteristics of persons who are most likely to experience poor physical health in later years. These persons have had poor health in earlier years, have experienced a critical recent event such as widowhood, and are dissatisfied with their current social activities.

Social and Health Profiles of Persons Perceiving a Negative Social Well-Being in Later Life

The social well-being (SWB) index measured in 1977 was used as a dependent variable in the AID analysis. The predictor trees of this analysis are presented in figure 8–3. A profile of individuals who had the highest or the lowest level of social well-being in 1977 can be summarized as follows:

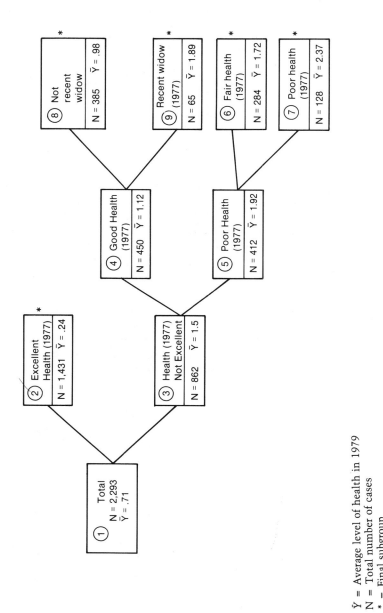

Ȳ = Average level of health in 1979
N = Total number of cases
* = Final subgroup

Figure 8–2. Predictor Trees for Automatic Interaction Detector (AID) Analysis of Health Index in 1979 by Selected Predictors

Group Identification	Profile	Mean SWB Index
Group 11	Unsatisfied with current activities and experienced a negative SWB in 1975	2.17 (lowest level)
Group 6	Very satisfied with current activities, positive SWB in 1975, and had annual family income more than $8,000	0.14 (highest level)

The SWB index in 1979 was analyzed by the same approach. We found that two important variables, the lagged SWB variable and income levels, made several splits of the total group into five final groups. Persons who had the worst level of SWB in 1979 were the members of group 9 ($\bar{Y}$ = 1.97), whereas persons who had an excellent rating of SWB in 1977 and earned an income more than $5,000 a year, had the best level of SWB ($\bar{Y}$ = .20) in 1979 (see figure 8–4).

Table 8–2
Automatic Interaction Detector Analysis of the Relative Contribution of Selected Sociodemographic Variables and Lagged Health and Social Well-Being (SWB) Variables in Explaining Variance in Social Well-Being (N = 2,293)

	Social Well-Being Index[a]	
	1977	1979
Predictors		
Lagged health variable	8.42	8.10
Lagged SWB variable	15.44	24.73
Age	0·07	0.06
Sex	0.02	0.01
Race	3.98	2.26
Recency of retirement	0.94	0.46
Recency of widowhood	1.12	0.34
Income levels	6.96	7.92
Participation in senior center activities	0.34	0.47
Dissatisfaction with present activities	15.63	9.99
Number of living children	1.56	0.86
R^2 (% variation explained)	32.90	34.00

[a]A composite index ranging from 0 (excellent) to 3 (poor) SEB was computed.

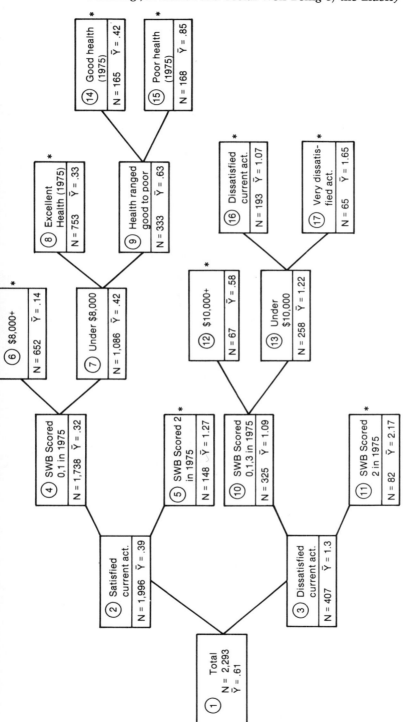

$\bar{Y}$ = Average level of social well-being in 1975
N = Total number of cases
* = Final group

Figure 8–3. Predictor Trees for Automatic Interaction Detector (AID) Analysis of the Social Well-Being (SWB) Index in 1977 by Selected Predictors

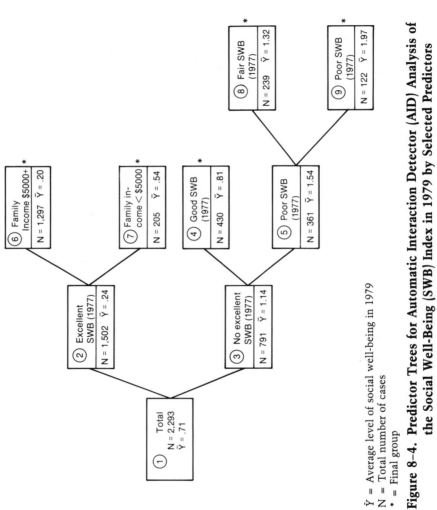

$\bar{Y}$ = Average level of social well-being in 1979
N = Total number of cases
* = Final group

Figure 8–4. Predictor Trees for Automatic Interaction Detector (AID) Analysis of the Social Well-Being (SWB) Index in 1979 by Selected Predictors

About one-third of the total variance in SWB scores can be accounted for by the eleven predictor variables, irrespective of the year
studied. A consistent profile of persons who were most likely to perceive
a negative SWB were those who had a poorer level of SWB in earlier
periods, earned less family income, and were more dissatisfied with
their present activities than others (table 8–2).

Validation of the Classification of Frailty Status

Several researchers have noted that classifications of well-being levels
by physical health and social well-being indicators may yield meaningful results in identifying service needs of the elderly [4, 5]. However, the
usefulness of the classification has to be demonstrated in terms of its
predictive as well as construct validity. For instance, in the present
study the level of frailty can be measured by cross-classifications of
physical health and social well-being levels, each well-being dimension
being dichotomized into good (scored 0–1) and poor (scored 2–3) levels.
This will make four broad categories of frailty: (1) not frail—sound physical health and good sense of social well-being; (2) minimally frail—
sound physical health and poor sense of social well-being; (3) moderately frail—poor physical health and good sense of well-being; and
(4) severely frail—poor in both physical and social well-being levels. We
can use the frailty status measured in 1977 to predict the utilization of
health services and the level of family income of the panel members in
1979. If this frailty classification can identify the differential in health
and socioeconomic consequences of the elderly, it should offer some
empirical evidence of its predictive validity.

Before we validate the frailty construct, illustrations of the profiles
or characteristics of the elderly classified in the four frailty groups are
needed. Of 2,293 panelists studied, the percentages for these four subgroups were 73.4 (not frail), 8.7 (minimally frail), 10.9 (moderately
frail), and 7.1 (severely frail). Detailed characteristics of older adults by
frailty status in 1977 are presented in table 8–3.

Several interesting differentials in frailty status are noted as follows.
First, age had no relevancy in differentiating persons in varying categories of frailty status. This has confirmed the fact that the traditional
concept of frailty associated with age is biased, if not incorrect. Thus,
frailty should be conceptualized as a phenomenon resulting from the
synergistic effect of poor physical health and a negative sense of social
well-being. Second, more males were either moderately or severely frail
as compared with females. Third, fewer whites appeared to be frail than

Table 8–3
Selected Characteristics of Older Adults in Frailty Status in 1977
(N = 2,293)

	Frailty Status			
Characteristics	*Not Frail*	*Minimal*	*Moderate*	*Severe*
Age (χ^2 = 10.6 with 15 d.f.)				
66	19.2	24.6	17.2	16.0
67	16.8	15.6	17.6	17.9
68	17.0	19.1	14.4	16.0
69	15.6	14.1	18.4	18.5
70	16.9	13.6	16.4	16.0
71	14.5	13.1	16.0	15.4
Sex (χ^2 = 10.8 with 3 d.f.)[a]				
Male	72.4	64.8	81.6	80.2
Female	27.6	35.2	18.4	19.8
Race (χ^2 = 78.7 with 3 d.f.)				
White	93.1	76.4	92.0	80.9
Nonwhite	6.9	23.6	8.0	19.1
Recency of retirement (χ^2 = 81.7 with 12 d.f.)[a]				
Not retired in 1977	10.3	4.5	3.5	1.2
Retired in 1977	36.2	36.7	23.2	31.5
Retired since 1975	31.9	36.2	52.0	51.2
Retired since 1973	21.3	22.1	20.8	14.8
Retired since 1971	0.3	0.5	0.4	1.2
Recency of widowhood (χ^2 = 38.9 with 9 d.f.)[a]				
Not widowed in 1977	79.2	62.8	81.5	71.0
Widowed in 1977	4.3	8.5	6.8	8.6
Widowed since 1975	17.3	24.6	10.0	15.4
Widowed since 1973	2.2	4.0	1.6	4.9
Income level (χ^2 = 230.5 with 18 d.f.)[a]				
Under $5,000	14.4	38.2	26.8	49.4
$5,000–7,999	15.1	22.1	13.2	17.3
$8,000–9,999	9.6	8.0	8.4	2.5
$10,000–14,999	15.8	5.5	14.8	3.1
$15,000–24,999	10.7	2.0	7.6	1.2
$25,000 plus	5.6	0.0	2.0	0.0
Unknown	28.8	24.1	27.2	26.5
Dissatisfaction with current activities (χ^2 = 709.6 with 9 d.f.)[a]				
Very satisfied	15.2	2.5	4.4	.6
Satisfied	77.0	64.3	56.4	30.9
Dissatisfied	7.5	26.1	26.0	30.9
Very dissatisfied	0.4	7.0	13.2	37.7
Number of living children (χ^2 = 35.9 with 12 d.f.)[a]				
None	20.6	14.1	20.8	12.3
One	18.6	17.1	16.4	17.9
Two	23.8	20.6	18.4	19.8
Three	16.0	17.6	16.8	13.6
Four or more	21.0	30.7	27.6	36.4

Note: Figures are column percentages.
[a]$p < .05$.

nonwhites. Fourth, about half of the severely or moderately frail had been retired since 1975. Fifth, recency of widowhood was significantly associated with frailty. Sixth, a disproportionate number of the severely frail had an income of less than $5,000 a year. Seventh, about 68.6 percent of the severely frail were dissatisfied with their current activities. Finally, the severely frail had a slightly larger proportion of persons with four or more living children than the other subgroups.

Frailty and Use of Physician Services. In order to validate the construct of frailty formulated in this study, we performed Multiple Classification Analysis, using the total number of physician contacts in 1978 as a dependent variable and frailty status and other sociodemographic characteristics as independent variables. Table 8–4 summarizes the results of the analysis. Of all the predictors included in the analysis, frailty status was the best predictor variable of physician contacts. The severely frail person had almost twice as many of physician contacts in 1978 as those who were not frail in 1977. Furthermore, individuals who were most likely to be identified as a high user of physician services were characterized as being severely frail, female, white, having been retired since 1971, not widowed, and earning an income of more than $25,000 a year.

Frailty and Family Income. The family income of the elderly in later life was estimated by using the frailty status, sociodemographic factors, and prior income levels as independent variables in the Multiple Classification Analysis. Table 8–5 shows that the lagged income variable was the most dominant predictor of family income in 1978. Frailty status ranked second relative to the other variables in determining family income. With everything being equal, income for the severely frail person was considerably lower than other categories of frailty status. More specifically, persons who had the lowest amount of family income can be characterized as (1) severely frail ($8,084); (2) aged sixty-nine ($9,787); (3) female ($9,188); (4) nonwhite ($9,250); (5) recently retired in 1977 ($9,933); (6) widowed since 1973 ($9,007); (8) earning income less than $5,000 in 1976 ($5,361).

In sum, a large portion of the variation in physician contacts and family income of the elderly panel can be accounted for by the frailty status. This provides some empirical proof of the validity of the frailty measure.

Conclusions

Despite our success in identifying social and health profiles of the frail elderly, it is important to recognize the limitations of our approach and

Table 8-4
Summary Statistics of Multiple Classification Analysis of Physician Contacts Made by the Study Panel in 1978
(N = 2,293)

	Annual Physician Contacts		
Predictors	*Unadjusted Mean*	*Adjusted Mean*	*Beta^2*
Frailty status in 1977			.031
Not frail	7.02	6.98	
Minimally	7.94	8.09	
Moderately	12.71	12.82	
Severely	13.51	13.63	
Age			.002
66	8.64	8.68	
67	7.63	7.59	
68	7.45	7.62	
69	8.12	7.95	
70	9.03	9.08	
71	8.15	8.11	
Sex			.000
Male	7.82	8.22	
Female	7.82	8.22	
Race			.000
White	8.15	8.20	
Nonwhite	8.50	8.04	
Recency of retirement			.000
Not retired	8.01	8.64	
Retired in 1977	8.11	8.28	
Retired since 1975	8.61	8.15	
Retired since 1973	7.57	7.83	
Retired since 1971	11.33	11.11	
Recency of widowhood			.000
Not widowed	8.35	8.33	
Widowed in 1977	7.78	7.16	
Widowed since 1975	7.64	7.94	
Widowed since 1973	7.54	7.41	
Income level in 1976			.002
Unknown	8.02	7.93	
Under $5,000	8.80	9.25	
$5,000-7,999	8.31	8.33	
$8,000-9,999	7.71	7.92	
$10,000-14,999	7.79	8.27	
$15,000-24,999	7.02	7.40	
$25,000 plus	9.83	10.66	
R^2			.034

Table 8–5
Summary Statistics of Multiple Classification Analysis of Total Family Income of the Study Panel in 1978
(N = 2,293)

Predictors	Total Family Income		Beta^2
	Unadjusted Mean	*Adjusted Mean*	
Frailty status in 1977			.009
Not frail	$12,066	$11,140	
Minimally	5,749	9,059	
Moderately	8,795	9,848	
Severely	4,571	8,084	
Age			.002
66	11,870	10,950	
67	11,796	11,070	
68	10,382	11,046	
69	9,772	9,787	
70	9,781	10,089	
71	9,666	10,518	
Sex			.007
Male	11,900	11,137	
Female	7,248	9,188	
Race			.002
White	11,004	10,714	
Nonwhite	6,215	9,250	
Recency of retirement			0.020
Not retired	19,767	15,842	
Retired in 1977	10,606	9,933	
Retired since 1975	8,906	10,293	
Retired since 1973	10,486	10,393	
Retired since 1971	6,182	11,322	
Recency of widowhood			0.002
Not widowed	12,004	10,815	
Widowed in 1977	8,843	10,486	
Widowed since 1975	6,024	9,913	
Widowed since 1973	6,287	9,007	
Income level in 1976			.377
Unknown	11,236	10,866	
Under $5,000	4,027	5,361	
$5,000–7,999	7,153	7,423	
$8,000–9,999	10,109	9,758	
$10,000–14,999	12,602	12,030	
$15,000–24,999	19,589	18,410	
$25,000 plus	39,302	37,382	
R^2			.510

its practical implications for program design and assessment in the aging field. Our assessment of the lagged effect of prior health and social well-being status on the well-being of the elderly assumes that other demographic, social, and role loss variables also play an important role in explaining the level of well-being of the elderly in the later years. That the elderly perceive a decline in physical functioning while cognizant of their changes in social adaptations or activities, or more specifically, that role losses and aging are concomitantly occurring in later life, are not fully taken into account. Although our findings suggest that the most predictive variable in utilization behavior (physician contacts) is the frailty status, this may nonetheless reflect the effect of a complex mixture of physical health and social well-being as an indicator of the need for care. Several aspects of program development to target the frail elderly must be considered.

First, information about personal characteristics and circumstances that may precipitate the risk of being a frail person in later life needs to be identified. This may improve our understanding of the etiology of frailty in the later years. Second, planning for the health or well-being of the elderly should focus on the development of appropriate social activities so that participation in satisfactory activities can reinforce an elder's positive feelings about his or her functional capacities. Third, to the extent that social activities are encouraged and facilitated, the elderly should be advised by clinicians or other health professionals to avert any physical or physiological abnormalities through the provision of primary preventive services. In other words, preventive health behavior should be fostered in the preretirement stage in ways that have implications for developing sound preventive practice.

Fourth, apart from any awareness on the elder's part, the development of incentives for maintaining good health practices may be necessary through the implementation of reduced health insurance premiums.

Fifth, the reduction of economic dependency of the frail elderly may be accomplished by introducing financial planning programs at the early stage of their retirement. For example, investment workshops, financial planning sessions, and personal counseling of financial managements can be incorporated in preretirement education programs so that the frail elderly can benefit from these services. The possible strategies in developing intergenerational economic supports toward aged kin should be considered in the social policy.

Finally, future research on the health and social consequences of role losses can build on the present findings to select a high risk group in a prospective study design so that the determinants of health and social well-being can be fully identified.

References

1. C. Coulten and A. Frost, "Use of Social and Health Services by the Elderly," *Journal of Health and Social Behavior* 23 (1982):330–339.

2. M.R. Haug, "Age and Medical Care Utilization Patterns," *Journal of Gerontology* 33 (1981):103–11.

3. T.T.H. Wan, "Use of Health Service by the Elderly in Low-Income Communities," *Milbank Memorial Fund Quarterly* 60 (1982):82–107.

4. T.T.H. Wan, B.G. Odell, and D.T. Lewis, *Promoting the Well-Being of the Elderly: A Community Diagnosis* (N.Y.: Haworth Press, 1982).

5. L.G. Branch, A. Jette, C. Evashwick, M. Palansky, G. Rose, and P. Dier, "Toward Understanding Elders' Health Services Utilization," *Journal of Community Health* 7 (1981):80–92.

6. T.T.H. Wan and G. Arling, "Differential Use of Health Services Among Disabled Elderly," *Research on Aging* 5 (1983):411–431.

7. F.D. Wolinsky and R.M. Coe, "Physician and Hospital Utilization Among Noninstitutionalized Elderly Adults: An Analysis of the Health Interview Survey," *Journal of Gerontology* 39 (1984):334–341.

8. S.D. Horn, "Measuring Severity of Illness: Comparisons Across Institutions," *American Journal of Public Health* 73 (1982):25–31.

9. T.T.H. Wan and S. Soifer, "A Multivariate Analysing of Physician Utilization," *Socio-Economic Planning Sciences* 9 (1975):229–237.

10. T.T.H. Wan and A.S. Yates, "Prediction of Dental Services Utilization: A Multivariate Approach," *Inquiry* 12 (1975):143–156.

11. J.N. Sonquist, E.L. Baker, and J.A. Morgan, *Searching for Structure (Alias AID–III)* (Ann Arbor: Institute for Social Research, University of Michigan, 1971).

12. R. Andersen, B. Smedby, and O.W. Anderson, *Medical Care Use in Sweden and the United States* (Chicago: University of Chicago Center for Health Administration Studies, 1970).

13. T.T.H. Wan and B. Livieratos, "Interpreting a General Index of Subjective Well-Being," *Milbank Memorial Fund Quarterly* 56 (1978):531–556.

9
Summary and Conclusions

B ased upon a panel of older males and females from the LRHS, a continuity model of well-being of the elderly was examined by the analysis of the linear structural relationships among preconditioned factors, role loss variables, coping responses, and health and social well-being indicators. The major findings of this study are summarized as follows:

First, elderly persons who had a favorable level of physical health in later life were those who experienced better health at the early stage of the aging process, irrespective of major role losses, economic status, and age. When retirement and widowhood were recent events, they had a negligible impact on the physical health of older adults in the later years. The effect of widowhood may be exaggerated if an individual's prior level of health is not considered. Intervention strategies should be established in the period in which optimal levels of health can be promoted through the establishment of healthy life styles such as having a balanced diet, exercising regularly, quitting cigarette smoking, and learning stress-management techniques.

Second, there is a distinct gender difference in perceptions of social well-being as related to role losses and other personal attributes of older adults. For the older males, the change in social well-being in later life was contingent upon their previous perceptions about their social, psychological, and economic circumstances, not the role loss experienced; whereas for the older females, a recency effect of retirement and a latency effect of widowhood on perceived social well-being were observed. This indicates that the life experience of older females is quite different from that of older males; therefore, it is imperative to develop sex-specific strategies in dealing with life-change events in later life. Furthermore, the development of early prevention of physical illness and negative perceptions of social well-being has an important role in the promotion of well-being of the elderly.

Third, retirement attitudes are relatively stable in the older population although wives' retirement attitudes are more stable than their husbands. Older couples are generally positive about retirement and especially so when both members of the couple are retired. For those who were negative about retirement, it was not the act of retiring that served as the impetus for such attitudes but rather the act of continuing to work that caused such couples to become more negative about retirement.

Fourth, the participatory life style developed in the preretirement stage has more influence on social participation than major role losses and other deteriorative changes experienced in old age. Continuity factors which depict this participatory life style, such as socioeconomic status, kin network size, and prior level of activities, are better predictors of participation than factors which reflect the experience of change such as widowhood and retirement. It is therefore suggested that the development of healthy life styles coupled with active participation in both formal and informal activities can help the elderly guard against the deterioration of social well-being in later life.

Fifth, identification of the frail elderly was accomplished by portraying their prior health and social well-being status. An index of frailty was developed and validated. We found that persons who were classified as severely frail (having a poor physical health and a negative perception of social well-being) were more frequent users of physician services and also had lower family incomes as compared with other persons. This index can serve as a useful screening measure of the need for care among the elderly.

The results of this study demonstrate the importance of prior levels of health and social well-being as preconditioned factors for the adjustment of the elderly in the later years. Although morbidity is more prevalent in the old than the young-old population, services should be geared to those with severe physical health disorders and economic limitations. Further, consideration must be given to the elderly who experience role losses within a specific time period since multiple events can significantly reduce their effectiveness in handling the distress resulting from long-term widowhood and involuntary retirement. In light of increasing budgetary cuts, the development of strategies for identifying a target population for services or interventions is deemed necessary.

Although retirement per se does not adversely affect the well-being of the elderly, there are retirees who are vulnerable to the potential of poor health. For instance, early retirees who retire for health reasons have been found to experience deteriorated health and decreased social activities in the later years. Both of these conditions may subject the elderly to a high risk of being functionally incapacitated. Thus, concerted efforts should be made to sustain or promote desirable social activities by strengthening existing interests rather than by implementing new ones, since neither leisure nor social activities show any significant changes following retirement [1, 2].

It is imperative to improve health and social services for the frail who are identified as having a poor physical health status and a negative sense of social well-being in the earlier period of retirement. The development of aging-related services should focus on primary prevention and foster active participation in activities in order to offset the social isolation resulting from the loss of spouse, shrinking friendship network, and decreased family interaction [3–5]. An increase in commitment by the public and private health sectors to "wellness care" for the elderly, such as early disease detection and health promotion programs, is urgently needed. Furthermore, social programs that can facilitate the development of positive social well-being should be instituted to include financing and subsidizing senior citizen activities. For those who may wish to return to work for economic or social reasons, public policies should be established to ensure equal opportunity for employment [6].

In conclusion, promoting the well-being of the elderly entails four basic elements—emphasizing the importance of primary prevention (for example, actions taken at the presymptomatic stage), making a rational selection of strategies from realistic options, correctly targeting the frail elderly for services, and establishing the priorities in the process of the implementation of programs. It is a challenging pursuit to develop a course of actions to handle the problems associated with aging. Public policy decision-makers should recognize the need for obtaining valid and reliable information about the health and social status of the elderly so that, based on the data generated from longitudinal studies, long-range planning for health and social services for the target population can be effectively formulated. Specific preventive programs that aim toward improving, maintaining, or lessening decline in the quality of life of older adults should be instituted. These include providing the elderly with preventive care in general practice [7], dietal and nutritional counseling [8], physical fitness activities [9], disease screening [10–11], and health education [12].

References

1. T.T.H. Wan, B.G. Odell, and D.T. Lewis, *Promoting the Well-Being of the Elderly: A Community Diagnosis* (N.Y.: Haworth Press, 1982).

2. A.I. Weiner and S.L. Hunt, "Retirees' Perceptions of Work and Leisure Meanings," *The Gerontologist* 21 (1981):444–446.

3. E.W. Bock and I.L. Webber, "Suicide Among the Elderly: Isolating Widowhood and Mitigating Alternatives," *Journal of Marriage and the Family* 34 (1972):24–31.

4. V. Karn, "Retirement Resorts in Britain—Successes and Failures," *The Gerontologist* 20 (1980):331–341.

5. T.T.H. Wan and B.G. Odell, "Major Role Losses and Social Participation of Older Males," *Research on Aging* 5 (1983):173–196.

6. L. Lowy, "Social Policies and Programs for the Elderly as Mechanisms of Prevention," in S. Simson, L.B. Wilson, J. Hermalin, and R. Hess (eds.), *Aging and Prevention* (N.Y.: Haworth Press, 1983).

7. D.W. Allen, "Preventive Care in General Practice," *Australian Family Physician* 8 (1979):118–133.

8. M. Bilderbeck, M. Holdsworth, R. Purves, and L. Davies, "Changing Good Habits Among 100 Elderly Men and Women in the United Kingdom," *Journal of Human Nutrition* 35 (1981):448–455.

9. J.F. Aloia, "Exercise and Skeletal Health," *Journal of American Geriatrics Society* 29 (1981):104–106.

10. W.E. Hale, R.G. Marks, and R.B. Stewart, "Screening for Hypertension in an Elderly Population: The Framingham Study," *Bulletin of the New York Academy of Medicine* 54 (1978):573–591.

11. J.D. Morris, "Geriatric Preventive Health Maintenance," *Journal of the American Geriatrics Society* 28 (1980):314–317.

12. P.A. Dinsmore, "A Health Education Program for Elderly Residents in the Community," *Nursing Clinics of North America* 14 (1979):585–593.

Annotated Bibliography

Part 1   Retirement and Well-Being for the Elderly

Part 2   Widowhood and Well-Being for the Elderly

Part 3   Retirement, Widowhood, and Well-Being for the Elderly

Part 4   Other Relevant Studies

Part 1
Retirement and Well-Being for the Elderly

Author(s) (date)	Analytic Technique/Sample Size/Study Design	Role Loss Measures	Major Hypotheses	Measure of Health	Findings
Anderson (1981)	Data used from U.S. Department of Labor force participation rates of males for 1970 and 1975 Study comparing relative impact of retirement and mortality on reduction in work force Double-decrement life table techniques and synthetic cohort employed in making comparisons of the probabilities of departure via retirement or mortality	Retirement			More males live to reirement with impact of mortality found to be negligible Median age of retirement occurring at a younger age, 60 years old in 1975 vs. 62 in 1970 Article discusses causes of rising number of retirees, such as declining infant mortality rates and the burden of these retirees on society due to their economic dependency
Atchley and Robinson (1982)	N = 1107, age = 50 years and older; longitudinal study to determine the effect of sociodemographic factors, including length of retirement, sex, and health on attitudes to retirement Data collected pre- and post-retirement. Zero order correlation and multivariate techniques used in analysis of data collected	Retirement	Attitudes become more negative just prior to retirement and people who have been retired longer have more negative attitudes than those who retired more recently		Perceived health and income adequacy were highly significant in predicting retirement attitudes Major disability is an important factor in unfavorable evaluation of postretirement years Attitude toward retirement is highly correlated with gender, health status, and income with men, those in good health and with adequate income levels having more positive attitudes in preretirement Postretirement attitudes correlated with health and income adequacy

Author	Methods	Topic	Finding	Topic	Comments
Bosse and Ekerdt (1981)	N = 581 males; interviewed in 1975 and again in 1978 via questionnaire to measure self-perceived levels of leisure activities. Since initial interview 125 had retired. Comparison made between retirees and continuing workers. Age (1978): retirees, median age 62.5; workers, median age 59.0. Age adjusted through covariance analysis; multiple regression analysis used to estimate effect of retirement status on leisure activities	Retirement	Retirement has a positive effect on perceived levels of leisure activities		Retirement does not produce perceptions of increased leisure time. Workers tend to overestimate positive aspects of retirement. Formal efforts to modify leisure pursuits of the elderly may be misplaced; encouragement of established activities may be preferable to new leisure activities
Burkhauser and Tolley (1978)	Discussion article; examines the economic incentives for early retirement	Retirement			Redistribution of social security funds to allow income maintenance to the elderly poor. Economic incentives of pension plans and SSI lead to less work at older age despite increase in mandatory retirement age
Casscells, et al. (1980)	N = 568 married white men. Comparison made between matched pairs of subjects to compute relative risk of retirees. Retrospective design biased in that wives of deceased subjects were respondents	Retirement	Retirement and coronary mortality may be linked	Mortality	Those who retired had 80% greater chance of coronary mortality than those who had not retired. Increased mortality may be due to the emotional stress caused by retirement

Part 1 (continued)

Author(s) (date)	Analytic Technique/Sample Size/Study Design	Role Loss Measures	Major Hypotheses	Measure of Health	Findings
Chirikos and Nestle (1981)	N = 3437, all males, ages 55–69 (1976) cross-sectional analysi of hours worked and disability level. Data from longitudinal study (1971–1976) correlated with cross-sectional data		Labor supply inversely related to impairment status Wages, hours worked, inversely related to degree of impairment	Self-reported disability or limitations in amount of work	Impairment status has an important effect in decision-making of males regarding work status Relationship between wages and impairments not as strong as found in previous studies
Ekerdt, Baden, Bosse, and Dibbs (1983)	N = 638; participants in Veteran's Administration Normative Aging Study. Prospective study using baseline and follow-up data on physical health provided by medical examinations to compare retirees (before and after retirement) and age peers still working Multiple regression techniques employed	Retirement	Retirement may not be detrimental to health	Medical examination	The changes in physical health did not differ significantly between those who retired and their working age peers. Also, types of retirement which are supposedly more difficulty to experience are not indicative of worse health
Ekerdt and Bosse (1982)	N = 498, all males; data taken from prospective study [Normative Aging Study] in 1975 and 1978. Age (1978): 56–67; median age 58.9 workers; 62.9 retirees Comparison between those who had retired since 1975 and those who remained workers to determine effect, if any, of retirement on health status Relative risk statistic used with age adjustment	Retirement		Self-perception of health status	Retirees and workers (in same age group) experience similar decline in self-reported health status Retirement due to disability, health problems affect evaluation of health status

Ekerdt, Bosse, and Goldie (1983)	N = 557, all males; prospective study of workers and retirees using data from Normative Aging Study of the Veterans Administration Age: retirees 53–73 with mean 63.0; workers 53–73 with mean 58.0 Results from responses to modified Cornell Medical Index collected at two different time points Methods: multiple regression techniques used to control for time between exams, age, T_1 results, retirement status, and presence of disability	Retirement	Retirement has negligible effect on health	Level of somatic complaints based on response to Cornell Medical Index	Level of somatic complaints do differ between retirees and workers of the same age group
Ekerdt, Bosse, and LoCastro (1983)	N = 263, all males; data obtained from Veterans Administration Normative Aging Study. Retirees who said that retirement had a good effect on health were compared with retirees who claimed no effect on health. Their response to a post-retirement questionnaire regarding relationship of retirement and health was compared to previous response taken preretirement for both groups Multiple regression used to relate role demand and job strain to appraisal of health during retirement	Retirement	Retrospective appraisals of improved health on retirement should be substantiated by data from longitudinal pre- and postretirement study	Health status	Retrospective claims of improved health not substantiated by longitudinal study Strength required on job not related to health status of retirees except in case of health-related retirement

Part 1 (continued)

Author(s) (date)	Analytic Technique/Sample Size/Study Design	Role Loss Measures	Major Hypotheses	Measure of Health	Findings
Ekerdt, Bosse and Mogey (1980)	N = 912, all males. Age (in 1975): 45–74 with mean age[5] 52.3 Data used from prospective Normative Aging Study. Subjects tested via questionnaire in 1965 and 1975 regarding age of planned and preferred retirement	Retirement			Preferred age of retirement is lower than expected age of retirement across all age cohorts studied Difference between preferred age and expected age of retirement decreases with age of cohort
Fillenbaum (1971)	N = 243; age = 25–54+. Subjects randomly selected nonprofessional employees of university and medical center. Questionnaire used to obtain information regarding job satisfaction, retirement plans, and beliefs. Health and difficulty in getting to work controlled in analyzing responses	Retirement	Those who are satisfied with their jobs will have a negative attitude toward retirement while those not satisfied will have positive attitude		Only possibility of achievement is related to retirement attitudes and only for males, whites, and the elderly Generally, job attitude is not associated with attitude toward retirement Job attitudes should influence retirement attitudes only when job has the central organizing position in an individual's life
George and Maddox (1977)	N = 58 males. Longitudinal data used to make comparison between retirement and adaptation during five-year period. Subjects were administered instruments prior to retirement and again five years later	Retirement			Little change in level of adaptation for subjects over 5-year period Social resources and socioeconomic status are important predictors of adaptation to retirement

	Methodology	Topic	Focus	Outcome	Findings
Glamser (1976)	Multivariate analysis techniques used to determine influence of variables on adaptation and retirement. N = 70 males; age = 60+; with mean age = 62. Mailed questionnaire used to determine relationship between various independent variables and attitude toward retirement. Zero order correlations of variables used to determine significance in retirement attitude and commitment to work. Multiple regression used to identify factors that determine retirement attitudes	Retirement	Attitude toward retirement is related to the type of retirement experience anticipated rather than concern with loss of work role		No significant relationship between commitment to work and attitude toward retirement. Support network, social activity level, knowledge of retirement, and previous periods of unemployment explained the majority of variance in retirement attitude
Gonzalez (1980)	Retrospective; N = 1,136 males; matched pair study [retired/not retired]. Age: 30–70. Data on occupation, medical history obtained from wives	Retirement	Effect of retirement in relation to fatal heart attack	Mortality	Retirement may lead to a higher chance of a fatal heart attack. Relative risk = 1.8. Findings only preliminary. Experimental problems, i.e., M. I. may follow retirement but need not be caused by retirement, and recall errors of some type may exist such as incomplete medical history

Part 1 (continued)

Author(s) (date)	Analytic Technique/Sample Size/Study Design	Role Loss Measures	Major Hypotheses	Measure of Health	Findings
Goudy (1981)	N = 5,091; age 58–63 (1969). Data taken from Social Security Administration Retirement History Study Sample. Initiated in 1969 with interviews conducted every two years. (Data from 1969 omitted because question on work expectations worded differently in subsequent years.) All males were married; females not living with spouses. No statistical analysis used in presentation of responses	Retirement	Those expecting to retire report later expectations or behavior more consistent with their initial expectations than those who do not expect to retire		Conclusions drawn from cross-sectional studies should not be used to formulate retirement/pension policies because work expectations change over time. Planning programs should be geared toward different types of users in order to reach all those that need to be served
Goudy, Powers, and Keith (1975)	N = 1,922; age ≥ 50. Workers in five occupational groups—self-employed professionals, owner-merchants, factory workers, and farmers—interviewed to determine work, income, social network, and attitudes toward work and retirement. Factor analysis used to determine three measures of attitudes toward retirement. Correlation coefficients used to determine relationship between work satisfaction and retirement attitudes	Retirement	Inverse relationship exists between work satisfaction and retirement attitude. Where work serves as a key organizing factor in worker's lives, relationship between retirement attitude and work satisfaction is inverse		Although some type of relationship between work satisfaction and retirement attitude exists, it remains unclear based on results of this study. Describes four types of relationships based on relationship between retirement attitude and work satisfaction and the need to plan retirement differently for each type

Author (Year)	Subject	Methodology	Hypotheses	Findings
Goudy, Powers, Keith, and Reger (1980)	Retirement	N = 1,152 males. Panel study with initial interview in 1964 and follow-up in 1974. Age = 50+ . Interviews conducted at two time points to elicit information regarding attitude toward retirement. Analysis of variance and paired t-tests used to examine data	Changes in individual retirement attitudes will be minor despite changes at societal level. Changes that do occur will be greater on the personal level. Retirement attitudes will differ by occupation with little difference within occupational groups over time. Those who continue to work will change to more negative attitude toward retirement; those who retire will move to more positive attitude	Change, either upward or downward, in retirement age was not significantly related to attitude toward retirement over time. As measured in this study, personal retirement attitudes changed less than societal attitudes. Difference in occupational groups exists over time but change over time with groups is noted. Employment status does affect retirement attitude
Gray (1983)	Retired or unemployed job seekers	N = 46; age = 50 or older. Longitudinal study of the effectiveness of an employment service geared toward elderly job seekers. Subjects were matched and randomly placed into either the experimental group which attended regular job club meetings or the control group which used normally available, staterun job placement services. Data collected over a 12-week period following the initial interview using personal and telephone interviews. Chi-square and analysis of variance performed		A job club program designed to improve job-seeking strategies of the old through self-help was found to be more effective than standard employment services used by the elderly. Need for local and national policies to improve job prospects for the elderly was discussed

Part 1 (continued)

Author(s) (date)	Analytic Technique/Sample Size/Study Design	Role Loss Measures	Major Hypotheses	Measure of Health	Findings
Hardy (1982)	N = 1,705; white males only (1975); age = 56–68 in 1975. Data used from the National Longitudinal Survey to examine factors influencing work force participation of subjects	Retirement			Retirement status is affected by amount and sources of retirement income Complete retirement associated with reporting health liminations and being covered by pensions and compulsory retirement as well as pension coverage only Being relatively well-educated (<65 years old) and being self-employed in high status jobs (≥65 years old) reduces probability of complete retirement Workers (65–68 years old) receiving income and benefits are much more likely to be self-employed or have low levels of job tenure and net assets
Haynes, McMichael, and Tyroler (1977)	N = 2,129; age = 56–64. Prospective study used to determine relationship between mortality and retirement process Case-control design used to test social factors' relationship with mortality during five years after retirement Data collected from medical, pension, and personal records with relative risk computed	Retirement (involuntary)	If retirement increases stress among those forced to retire, increased mortality would be expected during postretirement years Anticipation of retirement should increase mortality in workers during two years preceding retirement	Mortality rates	Modest evidence to support excess mortality after retirement as well as honeymoon and disenchantment phases of retirement No increase in mortality noted as retirement approaches. Effect of early retirement due to disability or illness questioned Low social status is associated with mortality during first three years of retirement

Study	Method	Topic	Hypotheses	Findings
Haynes, McMichael, and Tyroler (1978)	N = 3,971; prospective study used to compare normal retirees (N = 2,129) and early retirees (N = 1,842). Relationship between mortality and retirement process tested Data collected from medical, pension, and personal records with relative risk calculated based on expected mortality rates for working population	Retirement	If retirement is a stressful event for those forced to retire at age 65, mortality will be higher during the first five years after retirement If early retirement is taken because of bad health, mortality will be higher during first five years after retirement Those most likely to die after normal or early retirement will have low social status before leaving work force; have poor health during working career especially two years before retirement; experience less job satisfaction; and have less social support from family and others	Those more likely to die within five years of retirement have low social status before leaving work force, experience job dissatisfaction prior to leaving job, and have less social support from family and others
		Mortality rates		Mortality after early retirement is higher than expected and is related to poorer health status of this group Low social status associated with increased mortality for normal retirees. No relationship between low social status and early retirement found

Part 1 (continued)

Author(s) (date)	Analytic Technique/Sample Size/Study Design	Role Loss Measures	Major Hypotheses	Measure of Health	Findings
Hinds [1963]		Retirement			Provides overview of the impact of retirement on individuals (increasing percent of population ≥ 65 years old); compulsory retirement as defined by chronological age; cross-cultural differences in age of forced retirement; impact of health on decision to retire and postretirement years; and stages of retirement
Jacob (1978)	N = 30; 50% female; age 65-84 years old. Study of subjects who had returned to work after age 65. Comparison made between re-employed and unemployed (those interested in obtaining work but unable to do so) retirees. Reasons for returning to work, as well as how job obtained, were listed	Retirement			Those retirees who had re-entered the job market were of high morale compared to the unemployed group who felt rejected and morose. More jobs should be made available to retirees interested in working. More information should be made available to pre- and postretirees regarding job opportunities
Jaslow (1976)	N = 2,398, females only; age = 65 and older, with 71.7 mean age Cross-sectional study of the impact of work on female	Retirement	Older women still working have better morale than those who do not work (retirees and never-worked)	General health status, physical incapacity	Employed women had higher morale than nonworking women except for subjects with income >$5,000; then retirees had better morale

Reference	Methodology	Topic	Findings
	morale and health Comparison made between females who were still in the work force, retired or those who had never worked		Women who had never worked had lowest morale Employment found to be important because of financial advantage and possible psychological benefits of work
Karn (1980)	N = 1,000. Elderly who had migrated to two resorts were surveyed regarding their satisfaction with their move	Retirement	Retirees who migrated to resorts from the city were highly satisfied with move Reasons for dissatisfaction were isolation from old friends and family, especially children Need is stressed for improved social and health services for new elderly residents
McConnel and Deljavan (1983)	N = 4,004. Data were taken from the cross-sectional Consumer Expenditure Survey conducted by the Bureau of Labor Statistics. Using only households whose heads were 60 years and older, retired households (N = 2,100) and nonretired households (N = 1,904) were compared regarding consumption patterns Multivariate analysis used to determine significance of difference between these groups	Retirement	Retired households spent a larger portion of their budget on shelter, medical care, gifts, and contributions Retired households spend a larger proportion of income on medical care and have more out-of-pocket medical expenses Age was found to have a more significant impact on expenditures for the retired than the nonretired group

Part 1 (continued)

Author(s) (date)	Analytic Technique/Sample Size/Study Design	Role Loss Measures	Major Hypotheses	Measure of Health	Findings
McMahan and Ford (1955)	N = 4,230. Two groups of retired military officers were compared regarding survival ratio for 15-year period following retirement. Group 1 (N = 2,798) died during period 1925–1948. Group 2 (N = 1,432) retired during period 1925–1933. Rates computed for 3–5 year periods after retirement Chi-square used to test significance	Retirement	Survival rates are lower during first five years of retirement		Officers entering retirement at age 60 or older had higher survival ratio than those who retired at younger age No evidence to support hypothesis found
Martin and Doran (1966)	N = 604. Case-control study of retired and still-working males Comparison made between groups regarding presence and severity of illness. Age: 55–65 control group; ≥65 for cases Not longitudinal study. Pre- and post-retirement information based on interviews	Retirement		Physical health as measured by information obtained during interviews	Men over age 55 show steadily increasing incidence of serious illness until at or about retirement. Retirement shows decline in serious illness. Preretirement years similar for both cases and controls Compulsory retirement associated with reduction in incidence of serious illness

Moser (1974)	Discussion article	Retirement		Mandatory retirement seen as having negative impact on health and mortality and as being a waste of highly skilled elderly workers; call for abolishment of mandatory laws
				Discussion of family and society problems associated with increasingly elderly population
O'Rand (1982)	N = 5,350; males = 4,273 and females = 1,077 (all unmarried Data taken from the LRHS for years 1969 and 1971. Subjects compared to determine impact of various social and economic factors on post-retirement health	Retirement	Differences in life events prior to retirement will affect the impact of this role loss on post-retirement health assessment	Objective health, as measured by physical limitations and self-rated status	Women's self-perceived health status was negatively affected by retirement while men's was not; this is probably due to the economic disadvantage caused by retirement and the increased social isolation experienced by female retirees
	Independent variables: race, age, education, sex, number of children, location of job, job status, income (pre- and postretirement), level of impairment, marital status Dependent variable: self-rated health status				The relationship between retirement and health status is determined by the older individual's ability to maintain independent roles; both economic and social factors occurring prior to retirement influence this capacity for independence

Part 1 (continued)

Author(s) (date)	Analytic Technique/Sample Size/Study Design	Role Loss Measures	Major Hypotheses	Measure of Health	Findings
Palmore, Fillenbaum, and George (1984)	Data from six longitudinal studies were used to examine the consequences of retirement while controlling for preretirement characteristics: 1) the National Longitudinal Survey (NLS); 2) the Retirement History Study (RHS); 3) the Panel Study of Income Dynamics (SPID); 4) the Duke Second Longitudinal Study (DSLS); 5) the Duke Work and Retirement Study (DWRS); 6) the Ohio Longitudinal Study (OLS) Three measures of retirement were used in the analysis of data—objective, continuous and subjective—because the difference in measurement can affect the results Two-stage multiple regression analyses (ordinary least squares) used with measures of retirement being added at the second stage	Retirement	Retirement will have substantial effects on outcomes directly and necessarily linked to it such as income That it will usually have little or no long-term effects on indirect outcomes such as health and activities Early retirement will have more negative effects than on-time retirement		Only 50–75% of the difference in income between retired and working males is due to retirement because of the effect of preretirement characteristics Retirement has little, or no, effect on health or most attitude measures Retirement has little effect on changing levels of social activity. Initial level of activity is the strongest predictor of postretirement activity Early retirement found to have stronger effects on decreasing income and health

Palmore, and Fillenbaum (1982)	Data from three national and four local longitudinal studies were analyzed to identify predictors of retirement Four different measures of retirement used: objective retirement (occurring at age 65 or over), early retirement (ages under 65), age of retirement and amount of employment (from full-time worker to total retirement Multivariate analysis used to identify significant predictors of retirement as defined by the four measures	Retirement	Health, sociopsychological status in varying degrees by the seven different studies	Factors that increased the incentive or necessity of retirement (i.e., SES, age, pension availability) were stronger predictors of objective retirement Early retirement predicted by job attitudes and self-rated health status Age of retirement is influenced by SES, health, job characteristics, and attitude to work Hours worked are predicted by job characteristics, primarily self-employed, mandatory retirement, and industry of job location
Parnes (1981a)	N = 3,487, males only. Age = 45–69 in 1966 Data used from the National Longitudinal Survey conducted from 1966–1976. Information collected using face-to-face interviews (1966, 1967, 1969, 1971, and 1976), mailed questionnaires (1968), and telephone interviews (1973 and 1975) was used to determine factors influencing pre- and postretirement years, such as impairment level and availability of pension and disability benefits	Retirement	Various measures of health and functional limitations	Labor force participation rates decreased and work-limiting health problems increased during the years of the study Level of impairment directly affected labor force participation and earnings Although labor force participation rates declined for black and white males, blacks showed a higher rate of decline primarily due to the effects of lower educational attainment and increased availability of disability benefits

Part 1 (continued)

Author(s) (date)	Analytic Technique/Sample Size/Study Design	Role Loss Measures	Major Hypotheses	Measure of Health	Findings
Parnes (1981b)	N = 3,487 males. Age = 55–69 (in 1976) Longitudinal study (1966–1976) involving face-to-face interviews as well as telephone interviews and mailed questionnaires	Retirement			Impact of mandatory retirement policies is small; more men retire due to poor health than forced retirement Elimination of mandatory retirement age may not increase number of elderly in the work force, Changes in pension and policies, as well as work strategies, must be adopted to make working more desirable to the elderly than retirement
Parnes and Nestel (1981)	N = 1,584. Longitudinal study (1966–1976) of males with seven interviews during study Data used from 1976 interview with males who had retired during study. Age = 59–69 Comparison made between those who voluntarily retired for health reasons, and those forced into retirement	Retirement			Impact of mandatory retirement plans is negligible because of number of workers who choose to retire voluntarily or retire due to poor health Men who voluntarily retire are more satisfied with life than those who retired because of health problems or those forced to retire Increasing mandatory age of retirement will be of little use in increasing number of elderly in the work force; other policies must be developed for this goal to be obtained

Quinn (1981)	$N = 5,790$; age = 58–63. Data used from 1969 cross section of a longitudinal study administered by the Social Security Administration (1969–1972). Comparison made between self-employed ($N = 836$) and salaried workers ($N = 4,854$) to determine extent of partial retirement	Retirement	Abrupt retirement may be financially and psychologically damaging, and those with few institutional constraints are more likely to utilize a period of partial retirement	Partial retirement more likely among self-employed, and they work longer hours than salaried workers who may be partially retired
	Retirement status correlated with health, income, age, and existence of pension or social security benefits to determine influence of these factors on retirement. Multivariate analysis used to identify effects of these factors on retirement decision			Health status associated with retirement status; those with health limitations more likely to be fully retired for both self-employed and wage earners
				Both pension eligibility and net worth impact on retirement status
				Part-time situations should be made available to meet unmet needs of older workers
Roadburg (1981)	Respondents interviewed by final-year nursing students. Interviews included open-ended questions that included how they defined "work" and "leisure" and what work and leisure activities they took part in. Subjects lived in metro Nova Scotia, Canada, and included 111 men from 50–94 with a mean of 71.1 and 134 women from 51–94 with a mean of 71.8. $N = 245$	Retirement		Type of retirement (either voluntary or forced) influenced definition of leisure; those who were forced to retire defined it freedom to do "own things" while those who voluntarily retired viewed it as "enjoyment or fulfillment"

Part 1 (continued)

Author(s) (date)	Analytic Technique/Sample Size/Study Design	Role Loss Measures	Major Hypotheses	Measure of Health	Findings
Shapiro and Roos (1982)	N = 2,221. Longitudinal study of elderly workers (N = 630) and retirees (N = 1,581) noninstitutionalized Comparisons made between these groups to determine if differences in utilization of services exists between retirees and workers Personal interviews used to obtain information concerning sociodemographic characteristics, self-reported health status, life satisfaction and number of health problems. Medical records of physician visits and hospital stays provided measures of utilization T-test used to test significance between group means; chi-square to test difference in distribution across groups	Retirement		Self-assessed health status; health service utilization	Retirees found to assess health as lower and be less satisfied with life than employed elderly Despite positive association between health status and life satisfaction, retirees showed no greater use of health services than employed Difference in use is due to retired having higher level of serious illness; illness rather than retirement determines utilization Policies to increase availability of work for elderly to increase life satisfaction and standard of living
Skoglund (1979)	N = 603; age = 60–75. Cross-sectional study of Swedish workers. Data collected from preretirees (N = 262) and retirees (N = 341) to determine the impact of job orientation on attitudes to retirement and whether differences exist between the	Retirement	Sense of job deprivation would be associated with reluctance to retire, low occupational status, and, for retirees, working past retirement Job deprivation would be associated with work		Preretirees anticipate more regrets than retirees actually experience Missing work is significantly related to job orientation and reluctance to retire No significance shown between work attitude and occupational status or marital status

Author	Description	Topic	Measure	Comments	Findings
	expectations and realities of retirement Information collected on sociodemographic characteristics and attitude toward retirement analyzed using stepwise multiple regression techniques			orientation Checking for differences between preretirees' expectations and retirees' actual attitudes toward missing work	(except for "divorced" where significance was found)
Soumerai and Avorn (1983)	N = 55. Part-time employment offered to retirees. Comparison made between those who were given these jobs (N = 25) and controls (N = 20) who were not employed to determine impact of employment on retirees' health and life satisfaction	Retirement	Self-assessed physical and mental health		Elderly employed found to have experienced higher life satisfaction, physical, and mental health levels than the control group Physical and social activities increased for those employed Need to make jobs available to those elderly who may be interested in staying in work force
Stokes and Maddox (1967)	N = 138. Cross-sectional study of white collar (N = 85) and blue collar (N = 53) workers who were retired one year or less in 1960 Dependent variables: 1) adaptation to retirement as measured by level of satisfaction; 2) work satisfaction. Occupation prestige is independent variable	Retirement		Occupational prestige is inversely related to successful adaptation in retirement, when length of time retired is not controlled	Inverse relationship found between level of prestige and satisfaction with retirement White collar workers more likely to attribute intrinsic rewards to their previous work than blue collar workers

Part 1 (continued)

Author(s) (date)	Analytic Technique/Sample Size/Study Design	Role Loss Measures	Major Hypotheses	Measure of Health	Findings
	Chi-square test used to test significance between groups. Bi-serial correlations used to test relationship between length of retirement and level of satisfaction. Note: purposive sample rather than random selection done to include various occupational groups	Retirement	Attribution of intrinsic reward by an individual to his work will be directly related to occupational prestige. Work satisfaction will be inversely related to satisfaction with retirement when length of time in retirement is not controlled. When length of time retired is controlled, occupational prestige level and satisfaction in retirement tend to become directly related as time in retirement increases		Work satisfaction increases the probability of satisfaction in retirement for blue collar workers but has the opposite effect on white collar workers. Impact of time in retirement mixed; white collar workers show fairly constant satisfaction level until fifth year of retirement when level decreases; blue collar workers show decline in satisfaction with slight decrease in fifth year
Thompson (1973)	N = 1,589. Study based on data from personal interviews with male subjects of non-institutional U.S. population 65 years old and older. Age = 65–98 with mean of 73. Morals is dependent variable; work status is independent variable. Physical health, age, income, act as control variables	Retirement	Retired males exhibit lower morale than the employed when controlling for socio-demographic factors that are related to both employment status and morale	Self-assessed physical health and functional disability	Lower morale of retired is due to poorer health, lower income, and more advanced age rather than retirement itself

Thompson, Streib and Kosa (1960)	N = 1,559. Data from Cornell Study of Occupational Retirement used to compare retirees with those who remained in work force. Interviews conducted in 1952 when all subjects were employed and again in 1954 when 477 of the subjects had retired Comparison made between retired and still-employed with regards to personal adjustment as measured by life satisfaction and feelings of dejection and hopelessness	Retirement	Preretirement attitudes influence personal adjustment to retirement. Willing retirees no more likely to become dissatisfied or dejected than employed Retirement has negative effect on personal adjustment only insofar as it affects economic wherewithal (income adequacy and economic deprivation)
Weiner and Hunt (1981)	N = 130. Median age = 65.5. Study to examine specific meaning of work and leisure as perceived by residents of a Ft. Lauderdale retirement community Questionnaire developed to examine the meanings of these concepts	Retirement	There was a significant relationship between work and leisure concepts; retirees satisfied with past work life were generally satisfied with their present leisure life Subjects' scores were generally found to be independent of sex Workers in unskilled jobs who were now retired perceived their opportunities to experience status and leadership as being far less favorable than workers retired from the more prestigious jobs

Part 2
Widowhood and Well-Being for the Elderly

Author(s) (date)	Analytic Technique/Sample Size/Study Design	Role Loss Measures	Major Hypotheses	Measure of Health	Findings
Atchley (1975)	N = 902; age 70–79; 428 married males; 169 married females; 72 widowers; and 233 widows Mail questionnaire used Two occupational groups; retired clerical and service workers from Midwest telephone company and random sample of retire public school teachers Dependent variables: Z groups—social psychological and social	Widowed vs. married Widowers vs. widows		Social psychological status	Importance of economic supports and income adequacy For working class females, widowhood associated with income inadequacy which is associated with low auto use and low social participation. High level of loneliness and anxiety result Widowers are better off than widows except for age identity Widowhood produces stress in certain sociopsychological areas (age identification and loneliness) different from married people Schematic model shown for impact of widowhood
Bankoff (1983)	N = 98, white widows who admitted to still being grieving. Mean age = 52 years Mailed questionnaires used to obtain data regarding role of social support from parents as well as children and friends, on the psychological well-being of widows	Widowhood		Self-rated psychological well-being	As long as parents are living, they provide the most effective source of support to enhance psychological well-being For widows without living parents, support from widowed friends enhances well-being

	Multiple regression analysis was used to determine the effectiveness of the support from these various sources. One-way analysis of variance was used for subjects with no living parents, who received no support from parents and those who received strong parental support. Differences between widows receiving various levels of support were compared			Widowed shown to have higher suicide rates than married and widowers demonstrate a greater rate among widowed. The amount of social isolation the widowed experience contributes to the higher rates. Other relationships can diminish suicidal behavior
Bock and Webber (1972)	N = 2,544 elderly respondents and N = 188 suicides were compared using data from a survey (1959) on marital status; presence of relatives, and organizational memberships. Death certificates provided similar data for suicides. Suicide rates were computed for categories of elderly widowed and married	Widowhood	Widowed are more likely to commit suicide than are married, especially males due to the greater degree of isolation males experience Alternative relationships can alleviate isolation to some extent and decrease suicidal tendencies	
Chevan and Korson (1972)	N = 9,875 widowed; variables; age, race, sex, educational achievement, income, labor force status, ethnicity, place of residence, fertility, marriage, and living arrangements	Widowhood	The increase in the percentage of widowed living alone is due to changes which are not uniform in family norms governing living arrangements of the	All of the social and demographic variables were shown to have an effect on widowed living alone, and many diverse living arrangements were uncovered. Age, race, and sex were shown to have

Part 2 (continued)

Author(s) (date)	Analytic Technique/Sample Size/Study Design	Role Loss Measures	Major Hypotheses	Measure of Health	Findings
	Data provided by the one-in-a-thousand sample of the 1960 U.S. Census. Cross-sectional study provides comparisons between social and demographic variables and living arrangements as portrayed by percentages. However, limitations of the study are exclusion of kinship relations outside the immediate household, inability to directly measure attitudinal and health components, and the point-in-time assessment		widowed. Demographic and social factors impact the living arrangements of the widowed and are related to the spread of the conjugal family system		distinct influence on widowed living alone. Widowed with high income and high educational achievement more likely to live alone with income being the better indicator of living arrangement. Ethnicity impacts the type of living arrangement for the widowed, and foreign-born live alone less than native born Region and number of children also exert an influence on widowed living arrangements
Clayton (1974)	N = 90. Prospective study with subjects matched by age (N = 61 years old) and sex with control group Widowed persons interviewed by psychiatrist; control group interviewed by psychiatrist; nursing instructor, and medical student	Widowhood		Mental and physical health status	Widowed experience more symptoms associated with depression than control group Although both groups shared bad health during period of study, no difference in utilization of health services seen other than use of sleeping pills by widowed Widowed experienced certain physical symptoms—blurred

Author	Topic	Method	Findings
			vision, shortness of breath, palpitations—more than controls
			Males and females share certain symptoms of bereavement, but females experience more sleep disturbance than males Loss of interest and irritability more common in those whose spouses had prolonged illnesses
Clayton, Halikes and Maurice (1971)	Widowhood	Prospective study. N = 109—76 females; 33 males; white, widows or widowers, randomly selected from death certificates and obituaries Subjects interviewed in 1969 to assess mental and physical status, as well as social network and compared with subjects from 1968 study Chi-square test used	
Cleveland and Gianturco (1976)	Widowhood	Data from North Carolina marriage certificates (April 1, 1970, through March 31, 1971) listing widows and the 1970 U.S. census statistics on the widowed in North Carolina provided age-specific remarriage rates for widowed. Data from national mortality rates provided information on risk of mortality Interval distributions (time from widowhood to remarriage), remarriage rates, and mortality rates were combined to estimate the probability of eventual remarriage for the cross-sectional study	Remarriage is a desirable alternative to widowhood due to the factors of status drop for widows, isolation, loneliness, and other social problems associated with widowhood White men have the highest remarriage probability, especially age 45 and under. White women also have high remarriage probability under age 35, but after that point are much lower than white males. Among blacks, males demonstrated a higher probability of remarriage. Higher probabilities for remarriage are greatest for the younger widowed, but there are more among the older age groups due to the increased incidence of widowhood with age Distribution intervals are less for males than females and greater for blacks than whites

Part 2 (continued)

Author(s) (date)	Analytic Technique/Sample Size/Study Design	Role Loss Measures	Major Hypotheses	Measure of Health	Findings
Ferraro (1984)	Literature review on impact of widowhood on level of social participation with discussion of the methodological characteristics of various studies published since 1960	Widowhood	Study considers two theses on social adaptation to widowhood: a) decremental—role loss causes increasing social isolation; and b) compensation—reduced social activity in one area (caused by role loss) results in increased participation in another area		Although some decrease in social participation may occur after widowhood, it does not occur immediately after the loss of spouse; with the exception of parents-in-law, stability of social relationships is noted; also impact of decreased economic status and health may be greater predictors of change in social participation than widowhood
Ferraro, Mutran, and Barresi (1984)	N = 3,863. Data were used from the longitudinal Survey of Low-Income Aged and Disabled conducted by the Bureau of the Census in 1973 and 1974. Only the aged subsamples were used to obtain a married (N = 1,569) and widowed (N = 2,114) group. Because of the low-income level of the subjects, results not generalizable to entire elderly population, especially the wealthy elderly. Results can be generalized to widows, who have been found to be disproportionately poor. Comparison made between married and widowed regarding level of social participa-	Widowhood		Self-rated health status	Perceived health positively affects friendship support for widowed and married groups, but only in widowed group does friendship support affect perceived health For both groups, age negatively influences friendship support Income and education aid overall adjustment to widowhood Loss of spouse results in an immediate decrease in perceived health status; this is discontinued after approximately one year of widowhood After a few years of widowhood both widows and widowers experience a reintegration in friendship networks

tion and factors influencing their level of social integration				
Heyman and Gianturco (1973)	N = 41; 14 males and 27 females. Age 60-94 (in 1955); mean age = 72. Mean age of widowhood: females = 73.1 and males = 74.8. Prospective study over nine-year period with medical, psychological, and lab exams given as well as social history taken. Student t-tests used to test significance of difference in status before and after widowhood	Widowhood	Physical, psychological, and social health determined by physicians and other professionals	Subjects adapted well to bereavement with little significant change occurring after widowhood. This may be due to advanced age of subjects (80% 70 and over). Small significant change in attitudes to work and usefulness as well as overall attitude score
Lopata (1971)	Describes characteristics of widowhood, specifically for widows	Widowhood		Need for additional longitudinal studies to determine impact of widowhood and methods used to reorganize life. Need for programs to reduce isolation, loneliness of widows discussed
Maddison and Viola (1968)	N = 574 females: Boston widows [N = 132], Sydney widows [N = 243]; Boston married [N = 98], Sydney married [N = 101]. Widows selected from certificates of male (age ≤60) deaths 1964-65) in Boston and 1966 in Sydney	Widowhood	Self-reported health with emphasis on recent or greater degrees of health problems	Health deterioration may be more prevalent following bereavement. Widows showed a greater amount of physical and mental health deterioration than the control groups, and the Sydney widows had a greater degree of deterioration than the Boston widows. The greatest difference is that psychological symptoms are

Part 2 (continued)

Author(s) (date)	Analytic Technique/Sample Size/Study Design	Role Loss Measures	Major Hypotheses	Measure of Health	Findings
	Data on social and demographic characteristics in addition to self-reported health were provided by a questionnaire designed to highlight recent or increased health complaints. Comparisons of the matched cases (widows) and controls (married) provided by statistical analysis (chi-square)				demonstrated more markedly in widows than married
Morgan (1976)	N = 232 widowed and N = 363 married women aged 45–74. Data provided from interviews on marital status, self-reported health, current age, previous year's income, employment status, and mean interaction with family members as well as morale. Analysis of covariance used to assess the main effect of marital status on the dependent variable morale (represented by a six-item, factor-analyzed measure) controlling for the effects of the other variables. Analysis carried further to assess black, American-Mexican ethnic groups individually	Widowhood	Variables: health, income, age, family interaction, and employment status may mediate the relationship between widowhood and morale	Self-reported health	Poor health is associated with significantly lower morale among widowed. At higher ages, however, widowed have higher morale than married. When income and employment status are held constant, the impact of marital status is not significant. Family interaction has a positive impact on morale especially among Mexican-American widowed. Thus, factors other than widowhood may impact morale

Morgan (1983a)	N = 5,557. Data used from two waves of the LRHS. Comparison made between married males (N = 4,518), widows (N = 825), and widowers (N = 214) regarding differences in intergenerational financial support. Descriptive statistics and multivariate analysis used to explain observed pattern of 1975 support	Widowhood	Loss of spouse reduces the likelihood that the surviving parent will continue financial support to adult children. Intergenerational support is different for widows and widowers. Sociodemographic variables other than sex and widowhood affect likelihood of financial assistance to adult children	Widowhood does not alter the pattern of financial assistance that existed prior to the loss of spouse. Racial differences exist with nonwhites contributing more financial assistance despite economic strain caused by this action. Marital status and sex have no impact on provision of assistance. Higher annual income increases likelihood of assistance but its effect is small
Morgan (1983b)	N = 5,119. Data from LRHS (1969-1975) used to compare family interactions of married males (N = 4,293) with widowers (N = 225) and widows (N = 601). Widows were surviving spouses of original male subjects. Two measures of family contact were used: an average level of contact and total contact with relatives. Descriptive analysis used to compare married with widowed group. Multivariate regression and residualized change analysis were used to evaluate change in level of interaction over time	Widowhood		A decrease in family size of the widowed is the cause of a decrease in total family interaction reported in previous studies as well as this paper. Widows, however, see family members more frequently than when married, for widowers no change in frequency of family visits was found

Part 2 (continued)

Author(s) (date)	Analytic Technique/Sample Size/Study Design	Role Loss Measures	Major Hypotheses	Measure of Health	Findings
Mott and Haurin (1981)	N = 2,566 males. Longitudinal study of men under 65 years of age at time of death (N = 737), reference group of survivors from original study (N = 1,385), and wives of deceased subjects. Age = males 44–65 and females 30–44 Examines influence of sociodemographic variables on mortality, impact of declining health in years before death. Females studied to determine difference in circumstances pre- and postdeath of spouse	Widowhood			Health problem most significant predictor of death; when health controlled, those who are unemployed have higher risk of mortality Impact of death differs depending on length of illness of breadwinner Regardless of length of illness, real family income following widowhood decreases substantially
Parkes, (1964)	N = 44; age 38–81 with mean age = 60.2. Medical records of widows studied to determine difference in morbidity two years pre- and postdeath of husbands	Widowhood		Physical and psychological complaints as indicated by medical records	Morbidity as indicated by physician visits is highest during first six months following bereavement Both psychiatric and nonpsychiatric complaints increased after bereavement; psychiatric rates returned to prebereavement levels while nonpsychiatric rates remained elevated Psychiatric complaints found primarily for those under 64 years old; nonpsychiatric complaints among the elderly 65 and older

Reference	Topic	Sample/Method	Findings
Parkes, Benjamin and Fitzgerald (1969)	Widowhood	N = 4,486; age = 55 or older. Longitudinal study of widowers during nine-year period following wives' deaths. Rates for widowers compared with expected rates for married men in same age group	Increase in mortality of widowers during first six months noted: 40% higher than rate for married men of same age. After first six months, rate approximates that of married men
Pelham and Clark (1983)	Widowhood	N = 528; age = 65–90+ with average approximately 78. Data obtained from the California Senior Survey. Using subsample of low-income, noninstitutionalized widows residing in purposively chosen communities of California, comparisons were made between white (n = 331), black (N = 102), Hispanic (N = 49), and Asian (N = 46) widows. Data obtained via personal interviews. Descriptive statistics used to determine differences between racial/ethnic groups in sociodemographic factors, informal and formal support networks, and physical and psychological health status. Multivariate analysis used to examine relationship of racial/ethnic group and use of formal and informal services, and level of familial contact	Racial/ethnic differences exist in the living arrangements chosen; blacks and whites prefer to live alone, Asians and Hispanics with others. Living alone, level of dependency, and having children are related to familial contact. Living alone is inversely related to the level of contact. While all groups of elderly received informal support, the minorities—especially Hispanics—had a significantly higher level of support than whites

Part 2 (continued)

Author(s) (date)	Analytic Technique/Sample Size/Study Design	Role Loss Measures	Major Hypotheses	Measure of Health	Findings
Pollack (1961)	Discussion paper details psychological adaptation to death of significant other person and stages of the mourning process				Mourning seen as an ego-adaptive process involving reaction to the loss of "object" and readjustment to the external environment. The acute stage of mourning which follows the loss has several phases—shock, grief, pain, and initial stages of "letting go"—and is followed by the chronic stage where readaptation to life occurs. Response to shock of death of significant other varies in intensity based on suddenness of the loss and degree of preparation ego underwent prior to this loss. Mourning routinely involves depression and melancholia but the shock can be of such magnitude that serious somatic dysfunction can occur
Young, Benjamin, and Wallis (1963)	N = 4,486; age = 55 years or older. Study of widowers to determine effect of duration of widowhood on mortality. Rates for widowers compared with expected mortality rates for married males of the same age group	Widowhood		Mortality rate	Excess mortality in the first six months of widowhood observed with widowers having a 40% greater chance of death than married men. After the first six months, the rates drop back to normal

Part 3

Retirement, Widowhood, and Well-Being for the Elderly

Author(s) (date)	Analytic Technique/Sample Size/Study Design	Role Loss Measures	Major Hypotheses	Measure of Health	Findings
Beck (1982)	N = 2,248 males; age = 45–59 years old in 1966. Data used from the National Longitudinal Survey of Mature Men administered by Ohio State University and begun in 1966. Information through 1976 used for this study. Independent variables: work status, existence of health problems, and socioeconomic factors. Dependent variables: life happiness and life satisfaction. Method of analysis: logistic multiple regression and ordinary least squares regression	Retirement; widowhood		Number of self-reported health problems and in health status during three-year period	Health plays significant role in determining older people's happiness or life satisfaction. Income positively related to life satisfaction. "Recently widowed" has negative effect on life satisfaction. Poor or recent change in health had negative effect on evaluation of retirement experience. Men retiring close to expected age of retirement evaluated experience more positively than those who expected to retire later in life. Early retirement had negative effect on life satisfaction
Palmore, Cleveland, Nowlin, Ramm, and Siegler (1979)	N = 375. Data collected from longitudinal study conducted by Duke Center for the Study of Aging and Human Development at four time points between 1968–76. Age = 45–70 (in 1978). Analyzes the physical, psychological, and social impact of	Retirement; widowhood		Health status as determined by physical examination. Psychological status	Major medical events had most impact on physical adaptation with little change in psychosocial. Retirement most negative event with impact on psychosocial adaptation; physical effects noted for those with lower resources

Part 3 (continued)

Author(s) (date)	Analytic Technique/Sample Size/Study Design	Role Loss Measures	Major Hypotheses	Measure of Health	Findings
	five life events—retirement, widowhood, spouse's retirement, major medical problems, departure of last child from home Regression and analysis of variance used in analysis of results			via measures of personality and intelligence	Multiple events tended to cumulate effects especially on life satisfaction; better resources tended to mitigate negative effects
Pearlin and Lieberman (1979)	N = 2,299 original subjects; 1,106 follow-up survey. Age = 18–65. Longitudinal study with initial interview in 1972 and follow-up in 1976. Examines impact of sociodemographic characteristics and life strains Gamma coefficients used to determine significance of relationship between events (normative and nonnormative events and role changes) on psychological status Analysis of covariance used to determine whether event or aftermath of event explains variance in psychological status	Retirement; loss of spouse		Psychological status as anxiety and depression levels	Retirement produces little psychological strain Exiting work due to health reasons produces significant level of anxiety and depression Loss of spouse very distressful whether through separation, divorce, or death Psychological strain due to reaction to financial hardship, assumption of new role rather than role loss; quality of the experience determines level of psychological strain

Rowland (1977)	Literature review on impact of environmental events on the mortality of the elderly	Retirement; widowhood			Widowed, especially males, have a higher mortality rate during the first 6–12 months following their bereavement with rates declining toward level of married after this period Relocation is stressful even for the elderly and results in increased mortality for those in poor health. Providing support and increasing the elderly's familiarity with new surroundings reduces likelihood of death Studies inconclusive on impact of retirement on mortality because of relationship between poor health status and early retirement
Wan (1982)	A panel study, using data from the LRHS. A subsample of 5,884 older adults from four of the six waves of the LRHS data was analyzed by a prospective study design	Retirement; widowhood; other role changes	Life changes exert an impact on the health of older adults	Self-assessed health; life satisfaction; disability; use of health services	Widowhood is found to be the most important predictor of poor health. Retirement had no adverse effect on health when other demographic variables and prior health were simultaneously controlled in the panel analysis. The social support networks did mitigate the effect of role changes on health

Part 4
Retirement and Well-Being for the Elderly

Author(s) (date)	Analytic Technique/Sample Size/Study Design	Role Loss Measures	Major Hypotheses	Measure of Health	Findings
Blazer (1980)	N = 986; male and female, age 65-plus; black and white, noninstitutionalized Retrospective study Examines relationship between stressful life events (as indicated by life events score) and mental health functioning			Mental health status	Individuals with high life events score had increased risk of mental health dysfunction Health care seeking behavior is related to an increase in the number of life events experienced When contributing factors are controlled, relationship between mental health and life stress events is reduced (weakened) Life events, as measured by instrument used, may not be important risk factors to elderly
Burley (1982)	Data gathered during a 5-month period in the spring and summer of 1975. Participant observation and open-ended interview were the main data-gathering tools in (Ethiopia). Seventy-four were interviewed ranging from 19 to 62 years with a mean age of 34. Interview focused on respondents' attitudes toward others in both rural and urban populations and self-perceptions of social status and esteem				Work status, respect, environmental circumstances, and income act as motivating factors among elderly who migrate and can add to sense of well-being and life satisfaction

Carstenson and Cone (1983)	N = 60; age = 66-86; males = 23 (mean age 74.53), females = 32 (mean age 75.45). Five subjects did not indicate sex Two different measures of life satisfaction—Philadelphia Geriatric Center Morale Scale and Life Satisfaction Index–B—were correlated with three unrelated measures to determine their discriminant validity Correlations, means, standard deviations, were used to analyze the data obtained through mailed questionnaires (return rate approximately 50%)	Self-ratings of psychological well-being	The two measures of psychological well-being were highly correlated, but both tests were also significantly correlated with a measure of social desirability Consequently, these measures of psychological well-being may actually be measuring other factors making the relationship between age and psychological well-being unclear Need for further refinement of measures is noted
Chiriboga (1982)	N = 216. Four groups undergoing events previously identified as stressful were selected for this longitudinal (5 years) study: high school seniors (N = 52), newlyweds (N = 50), parents facing an "empty nest" (N = 54), and those facing retirement (N = 60) Data collected three times during the study, two and five years after baseline information collected (1969) Information collected regarding stress reported in association with life events, emotional and psychological status	Psychological symptoms	For both sexes, highly stressed subjects had lower levels of satisfaction although highly stressed middle-aged mothers reported more positive emotions Number of symptoms reported declined over time but varied according to sex and group; highly stressed retired females showed increase in number of symptoms during last two measurements while highly stressed newlywed females showed increase in number of symptoms during first two measurements. Highly stressed retired males

Part 4 (continued)

Author(s) (date)	Analytic Technique/Sample Size/Study Design	Role Loss Measures	Major Hypotheses	Measure of Health	Findings
					showed greatest decline over time; no decline noted for high school or middle-aged stressed males
Cockerham, Sharp, and Wilcox (1983)	N = 660; age = 18 and older with mean age of 45. Study comparing aged (60 or older) with younger groups (18–60) regarding perceived health status Data collected via telephone interviews regarding socio-demographic characteristics and number of symptoms experienced Multiple regression used to control for effect of education and number of symptoms; correlation coefficients, means, and standard deviation used in analysis of data		Older people tend to see their health as better than others of their age	Self-perceived health status	Number of symptoms is strongest predictor of perceived health status followed by age, education, and race Aged found to have a more positively perceived health status than younger groups; although aged with less education experience more symptoms and lower health status No significance between widowhood and health status
Coyne, Aldwin, and Lazarus (1981)	N = 89; age: 45–64, all whites. One-year long study of stress and coping Comparison between depressed and nondepressed based on responses to self-reported questionnaires and information obtained through series of interviews			Level of depression; mental health status	Depressed need more information in order to make decisions; engage in more wishful thinking and seek emotional and informational support in coping

Ferraro (1980)	N = 3,402. Data from survey of low-income aged in U.S.; 63% of subjects were female; 89% were white. Mean education level = 8.45 years Independent variables: education, sex, age, disability level, number of illnesses Dependent variables: health status based on response to questionnaires Correlation and regression used to determine relationship between independent and dependent variables. T-tests used to compare age groups		Self-reported health status	Disability and number of illnesses related to aged's self-reported health status; therefore, self-rating measures can be used Self-ratings of health affected by sociodemographic factors such as educational level Old-old (75+) tend to report better health status than old (64–75) despite higher level of disability and number of illnesses
Fillenbaum (1979)	N = 998. Institutionalized elderly [N = 61, males = 23; females = 38; mean age = 80] Compared with noninstitutionalized elderly [N = 937; males = 348; females = 589; mean age = 73) to determine health status	Institutionalized elderly will have higher degree of health problems than noninstitutionalized	Self-reported health status and objective health measures	Self-reported status reflects actual health state among noninstitutionalized Sex differences influence self-reported health

Part 4 (continued)

Author(s) (date)	Analytic Technique/Sample Size/Study Design	Role Loss Measures	Major Hypotheses	Measure of Health	Findings
Gutman and Herbert (1976)	Subjects: 96 males ranging from 22–94 years. But only those 60 and over were used in the survey [N = 81]; 84.37% of them were 60 and over. Among those, average age was 77.93; 62.96% had some degree of confusion while 70.38% were nonambulatory. These figures were over a five-year period. Procedure: study was conducted in two stages over a 21-month period. First stage—document actual transfer procedure as well as all efforts on part of staff to prevent or alleviate relocation stress. Second stage—21 months after relocation obtaining data on mortality of relocation population to see how transfer affected their lives				No increase in mortality noted 3 months to 21 months following relocation. Ambulatory elderly showed significantly higher rate of mortality than nonambulatory patients in subjects; control groups showed opposite results and so do results of previous studies. Relocation of elderly if efficient and patients are well-informed and prepared need not cause increased mortality
Kasl, Gore, and Cobb (1975)	N = 94 males, age 35–60. Longitudinal study, unemployed matched with control group of continuously employed men. Study conducted in five phases; phase one,	Unemployment due to plant closing		Mental and physical based on interviews and lab work	Differences found in cases between urban and rural setting; support network of rural community seen as being the main reason for difference. Younger, better-educated initi-

	pre-plant closing, to phase five, two years after plant closing. Nurses interviewed subjects as well as physically examined (including blood and urine tests). Health diary maintained by subjects for 14-day period during each phase Comparisons made between control and case groups regarding effect of unemployment on health status, perceived disability, and illness behavior	ally had higher number of "days complaints" than older, poorly educated but this relationship reversed by phase five Period of anticipation can be as stressful as event being anticipated
Markides (1983)	N = 338. Longitudinal study (initial interview in 1976 with follow-up in 1981) of Mexican-American and Anglo elderly. Mean age = 69.8 (in 1976). Church attendance, self-rated religiosity, and practice of private prayer were used to determine whether religiosity increases with age and if this variable affects life satisfaction Means test, simple and multiple regression, were used to analyze the data collected. The two groups were analyzed separately in all cases	Effect of religiosity increases with age Religiosity is highly associated with life satisfaction Church attendance showed small but significant decline for Mexican-American; no change noted for Anglos Self-rated religiosity increased for both groups Mixed support found for association between religiosity and life satisfaction. Church attendance important for both groups but may serve integrative rather than spiritual function Effect of life satisfaction increases with age; private prayer for Mexican-Americans and church attendance for Anglos increased significant over time

Part 4 (continued)

Author(s) (date)	Analytic Technique/Sample Size/Study Design	Role Loss Measures	Major Hypotheses	Measure of Health	Findings
Markides and Martin (1979)	N = 480; age = 60 and older. Cross-sectional study of elderly Mexican-American (70%) and Anglos (30%) in Texas. Interviews conducted to determine effect of socio-demographic variables on health status Path analysis model developed which indicates interrelation of variables		Health index will have direct negative effect on self-rated health Income and education will have direct positive effect on self-rated health and indirect positive effect on the health index Age, female, and Mexican-American will have direct negative effect on self-rating and indirect negative effect on health index	Self-assessed health status, number and seriousness of health problems (health index), and degree of confinement to bed due to health	Health index greatest predictor of self-health ratings Age has indirect effect on self-assessed health through health index; elderly persons' higher scores in health index which caused lower self-reported health status Elderly of lower socioeconomic status (SES) tend to perceive themselves as having poorer health than persons of high SES
Morris, Wolf, and Klerman (1975)	N = 89, long-term institutionalized patients (two or more years); age = 20-86 with 53 median. Females = 49%; whites = 94% Subjects administered three separate instruments that measure morale and depression during two time points, 15 weeks apart Factor analysis and pairwise correlation used to develop a single instrument to measure depression and morale of elderly			Mental health status	Seven sets of items were found as common themes in the three instruments: 1) self-satisfaction; 2) life progression; 3) impaired thinking; 4) dejection; 5) guilt; 6) tranquility; and 7) agitation Pooled scale (segments from three measurements) seen as more reliable measure with cross-disciplinary uses

	Method	Variables	Findings
	Instruments tested were 1) Philadelphia Geriatric Center Morale Scale; 2) Gardner-Hetznecker Sign and Symptom Check List; and 3)Zung Self-Rating Depression Scale		
Mossey and Shapiro (1982)	N = 3,128; age = 65 and older in 1971, male/female evenly represented. Longitudinal study: self-rated health status obtained during interview in 1971. Objective health status determined from claims data or information obtained from subjects for year prior to study. Mortality measured for two time periods (1971–73) and (1974–77). Sociodemographic characteristics and life satisfaction score determined in 1971 interview. Analysis of self-rated health and stage of mortality while controlling for objective health and other independent variables was done using log linear and multiple logistic risk models.	Subjective and objective (physician) ratings of health	Self-rated health is a predictor of mortality. Risk of mortality approximately 2.8 times higher in those who rate health as poor than those who rate health as excellent. Self-rated health is second only to age in predicting of *early* mortality and is strongest predictor of *late* mortality. Relationship of self-rated health is independent of subjects' level of objective health
Osborn (1973)	N = 582. Age = 60–64. Longitudinal study using self-reported sociodemographic and health information of married males	Self-reported health status	Influence of social rank on self-reported morbidity varies with degree of severity of chronic illness; for those with no reported illness,

Part 4 (continued)

Author(s) (date)	Analytic Technique/Sample Size/Study Design	Role Loss Measures	Major Hypotheses	Measure of Health	Findings
	Attempts to determine relationship between social rank and morbidity. Chi-square test used to test significance. Modification of Pearsonian Contingency Coefficient used to test strength of significant associations				for those with no reported illness, influence of social rank is slight while among those with serious illness more individuals at the lowest income-education level rate themselves in poor health
Patrick (1980)	Discussion article on impact of health of the elderly on their migration			Monotonic—ranging from excellent, without illness, through various stages to death	Two types of migration: 1) migration in good health, such as the Sun Belt; 2) migration in bad health, to long-term nursing facilities or nearer relatives. Policy implications due to effect of migration on resource allocations: 1) should attempt to reduce impact of bad health, as through nutrition programs or home health aids; and 2) should reduce impact of increasingly elderly population on communities where they immigrate
Roos and Shapiro (1981)	N = 4,558. Longitudinal study of both institutionalized and noninstitutionalized elderly from 1970 to 1972. Interviews conducted in 1971			Self-perceived health status; physician	Elderly as a group are not high users of physician and hospital visits; small proportion of elderly account

Author/Year	Description	Variable	Findings
	were linked with physician visits and hospital contacts during 12 months pre- and postinterview. Examines relationship between utilization and sociodemographic factors. Ambulatory visits as well as total days in hospital used as measures of utilization	and hospital utilization rates	for large share of services used. Poor self-perceived health status number of health problems, and low income are associated with utilization. Need for additional research to determine differences between high users of services and their peers in order to implement policies to affect their use patterns
Rosencranz and Pihlblad (1970)	N = 1,700; age = 65 and older. Females = 1,035 (3/4 were widows); males = 665 (1/4 were widowed) Health index constructed based on weighted scores of subjects' responses to list of 40 ailments or medical conditions. Index divided into five ordinal classes and was correlated with self-perceived health status and functional capabilities to ascertain validity and accuracy of index as a measure of health status in the elderly	Self-perceived physical health	Score on index closely related to self-reported health status. Bodily impairment and physical limitation increases with decline in health as indicated by Health Index
Tissue (1972)	N = 256. Longitudinal study of elderly welfare recipients, noninstitutionalized during initial interview. Median age = 68; males = 111; females = 145. Second interview one year later	Self-assessed health status	Self-rated health are most closely associated with subjective and objective health rather than morale or self-image of the subjects

Part 4 (continued)

Author(s) (date)	Analytic Technique/Sample Size/Study Design	Role Loss Measures	Major Hypotheses	Measure of Health	Findings
	Response to interview questions on morale, response to aging, physical health, and subjective health status used to determine reliability of self-ratings by the elderly				
Usui, Keil, and Phillips (1983)	N = 657. Examines racial differences in life satisfaction between noninstitutionalized black (N = 219) and white (N = 438) elderly Sociodemographic factors and self-reported physical impairment were independent variables; life satisfaction the dependent variable Emphasis of paper is primarily methodological, rather than simply comparing results of one group with another; regression analyses using interaction terms are used				Without use of interaction terms, racial differences exist. Physical impairment, income, and formal and informal social participation are significant variables for whites. For blacks only physical and formal social participation show significance Using interaction terms, only physical impairment is significant with other variables having similar effects for both races
Vaillant (1979)	205 men; longitudinal study		Effects of mental health on physical health		Good mental health retards midlife deterioration in physical health

Wan, Odell, and Lewis (1982)	A community survey of 1,182 elderly residents in Baltimore County, Maryland, was conducted to assess the service needs and the well-being of the elderly	Functional capacities; self-reported health; disability; instrumental activities of daily living	Most of the needs of the study population were being met. Based upon a classification of health and socioeconomic status, the frailty status was determined. The planning and intervention strategies were recommended to target on the frail elderly

Bibliography

Anderson, T.B., "The Dependent Elderly Population," *Research on Aging* 13 (1981):311–324.

Atchley, R.C., "Dimensions of Widowhood in Later Life," *The Gerontologist* 15 (1975):175–178.

Atchley, R.C., and J.L. Robinson, "Attitudes Toward Retirement and Distance from the Event," *Research on Aging* 4 (1982):299–313.

Bankoff, E.A., "Aged Parents and their Widowed Daughters: A Support Relationship," *Journal of Gerontology* 38 (1983):226–230.

Beck, S.H., "Adjustment to and Satisfaction with Retirement," *Journal of Gerontology* 37 (1982):616–624.

Bock, E.W., and I.L. Webber, "Suicide among the Elderly: Isolating Widowhood and Mitigating Alternatives," *Journal of Marriage and the Family* 34 (1972): 24–31.

Bosse, R., and D.J. Ekerdt, "Change in Self-Perception of Leisure Activities with Retirement," *The Gerontologist* 21 (1981):650–654.

Burkhauser, R.V., and G.S. Tolley, "Older Americans and Market Work," *The Gerontologist* 18 (1978):449–453.

Casscells, W., D. Evans, R.A. DeSilva, J.E. Davies, C.H. Hennekens, B. Rosener, B. Lown, and M.J. Jesse, "Retirement and Coronary Mortality," *The Lancet* 1(8181) (1980):1288–1289.

Chevan, A., and J.H. Korson, "The Widowed Who Live Alone: An Examination of Social and Demographic Factors," *Social Forces* 51 (1972):45–53.

Clayton, P.J., "Mortality and Morbidity in the First Year of Widowhood," *Archives of General Psychiatry* 30 (1974):747–750.

Clayton, P., J.A. Halikes, and W.L. Maurice, "The Bereavement of the Widowed," *Diseases of the Nervous System* 32 (1971):597–604.

Cleveland, W.P., and D.T. Gianturco, "Remarriage Probability After Widowhood: A Retrospective Method," *Journal of Gerontology* 31 (1976):99–103.

Ekerdt, D.J., L. Baden, R. Bosse, and E. Dibbs, "The Effect of Retirement on Physical Health," *American Journal of Public Health* 73 (1983):779–783.

Ekerdt, D.J., and R. Bosse, "Change in Self-Reported Health and Retirement," *International Journal of Aging and Human Development* 15 (1982):213–223.

Ekerdt, D.J., R. Bosse, and C. Goldie, "The Effect of Retirement on Somatic Complaints," *Journal of Psychosomatic Research* 27 (1983):61–67.

Ekerdt, D.J., R. Bosse, and J. LoCastro, "Claims that Retirement Improves Health," *Journal of Gerontology* 38 (1983):231–236.

Ekerdt, D.J., R. Bosse, and J.M. Mogey, "Concurrent Change in Planned and Preferred Age for Retirement," *Journal of Gerontology* 35 (1980):232–240.

Ferraro, K.F., "Widowhood and Social Participation in Later Life: Isolation or Compensation?," *Research on Aging* 6 (1984):451–468.

Ferraro, K.F., E. Mutran, and C.M. Barresi, "Widowhood, Health, and Friendship Support in Later Life," *Journal of Health and Social Behavior* 25 (1984): 246–259.

Fillenbaum, G.G., "On the Relation Between Attitude to Work and Attitude to Retirement," *Journal of Gerontology* 26 (1971):244–248.

George, L.K., and G.L. Maddox, "Subjective Adaptation to Loss of the Work Role: A Longitudinal Study," *Journal of Gerontology* 32 (1977):456–462.

Glamser, F.D., "Determinants of a Positive Attitude Toward Retirement," *Journal of Gerontology* 31 (1976):104–107.

Gonzalez, E.R., "Retiring May Predispose to Fatal Heart Attack," *Journal of the American Medical Association* 243 (1980):13–14.

Goudy, W.J., "Changing Work Expectations: Findings from the Retirement History Study," *The Gerontologist* 21 (1981):644–649.

Goudy, W.J., E.A. Powers, and P.M. Keith, "Work and Retirement: A Test of Attitudinal Relationships," *Journal of Gerontology* 30 (1975):193–198.

Goudy, W.J., E.A. Powers, P.M. Keith, and R.A. Reger, "Changes in Attitudes Toward Retirement: Evidence from a Panel Study of Older Males," *Journal of Gerontology* 35 (1980):942–948.

Gray, D., "A Job Club for Older Job Seekers: An Experimental Evaluation," *Journal of Gerontology* 38 (1983):363–368.

Hardy, M.A., "Job Characteristics and Health: Differential Impact on Benefit Entitlement," *Research on Aging* 4 (1982):457–478.

Haynes, S.G., A.J. McMichael, and H.A. Tyroler, "The Relationship of Normal Involuntary Retirement to Early Mortality Among U.S. Rubber Workers," *Social Science and Medicine* 11 (1977):105–114.

———, "Survival After Early and Normal Retirement," *Journal of Gerontology* 33 (1978):269–278.

Heyman, D.K., and D.T. Gianturco, "Long-Term Adaptation by the Elderly to Bereavement," *Journal of Gerontology* 28 (1973):359–362.

Hinds, S.W., "The Personal and Socio-Medical Aspects of Retirement," *Royal Society of Health Journal* 83 (1963):281–285.

Jacob, R.H., "Reemployment and Unemployment in Old Age," *Journal of Geriatric Psychiatry* 11 (1978):78–80.

Jaslow, P., "Employment, Retirement, and Morale Among Older Women," *Journal of Gerontology* 31 (1976):212–218.

Karn, V., "Retirement Resorts in Britain—Successes and Failures," *The Gerontologist* 20 (1980):331–341.

Lopata, H.Z., "Widows as a Minority Group," *The Gerontologist* 11 (1971): 67–77.

McConnel, C.E., and F. Deljavan, "Consumption Patterns of the Retired Household," *Journal of Gerontology* 38 (1983):480–490.

McMahan, C.A., and T.R. Ford, "Surviving the First Five Years of Retirement," *Journal of Gerontology* 10 (1955):212–215.

Maddison, D., and A. Viola, "The Health of Widows in the Year Following Bereavement," *Journal of Psychosomatic Research* 12 (1968):297–306.

Martin, J., and A. Doran, "Evidence Concerning the Relationship Between Health and Retirement," *Sociological Review* 14 (1966):329–343.

Morgan, L.A., "A Re-Examination of Widowhood and Morale," *Journal of Gerontology* 31 (1976):687–695.

——, "Changes in Family Interaction Following Widowhood," *Journal of Marriage and the Family* 46 (1983):323–332.

——, "Intergenerational Economic Assistance to Children: The Case of Widows and Widowers," *Journal of Gerontology* 38 (1983):725–731.

Moser, R.H., "The Old Folks at Home: Variations on a Theme," *Journal of the American Medical Association* 230 (1974):1311–1314.

Mott, F.L., and R.J. Haurin, "The Impact of Health Problems and Mortality on Family Well-Being," in H.S. Parnes (ed.), *Work and Retirement: A Longitudinal Study of Men* (Cambridge, Mass.: MIT Press, 1981).

O'Rand, A.M., "Loss of Work Role and Subjective Health Assessment in Later Life Among Men and Unmarried Women," in A.C. Kerckhoff (ed.), *Research in the Sociology of Education and Socialization*, Vol. 5 (Greenwich, Conn.: JAI Press, 1982).

Palmore, E.B., W.P. Cleveland, J.B. Nowlin, D.F. Ramm, and I. Siegler, "Stress and Adaptation in Later Life," *Journal of Gerontology* 34 (1979):841–851.

Palmore, E.B., G.G. Fillenbaum, and L.K. George, "Consequences of Retirement," *Journal of Gerontology* 39 (1984):109–116.

Palmore, E.B., L.K. George, and G.G. Fillenbaum, "Predictors of Retirement," *Journal of Gerontology* 37 (1982):733–742.

Parkes, C.M., "Effects of Bereavement on Physical and Mental Health—A Study of the Medical Records of Widows," *British Journal of Medicine* 2 (1964): 274–279.

Parkes, C.M., B. Benjamin, and R.G. Fitzgerald, "Broken Heart: A Statistical Study of Increased Mortality Among Widowers," *British Medical Journal* 1 (1969):740–743.

Parnes, H.S., "From the Middle to the Later Years, Longitudinal Studies of the Pre- and Post-Retirement Experiences of Men," *Research on Aging* 3 (1981): 387–402.

—— (ed.), *Work and Retirement: A Longitudinal Study of Men*, (Cambridge, Mass.: MIT Press, 1981).

Parnes, H.S., and G. Nestel, "The Retirement Experience," in H.S. Parnes (ed.), *Work and Retirement: A Longitudinal Study of Men* (Cambridge, Mass.: MIT Press, 1981).

Pearlin, L.I., and M.A. Lieberman, "Social Sources of Emotional Distress," *Research in Community and Mental Health* 1 (1979):217–248.

Pelham, A.O., and W.F. Clark, "Widowhood Among Low-Income Ethnic Minorities in California." Paper presented at the 111th Annual Meeting of the American Public Health Association, Dallas, November 1983.

Pollack, G.H., "Mourning and Adaptation," *International Journal of Psycho-*

analysis 42 (1961):341–361.

Quinn, J.F., "The Extent and Correlates of Partial Retirement," *The Gerontologist* 21 (1981):634–643.

Roadburg, A., "Perceptions of Work and Leisure Among the Elderly," *The Gerontologist* 21 (1981):142–145.

Rowland, K.F., "Environmental Events Predicting Death for the Elderly," *Psychological Bulletin* 84 (1977):349–372.

Shapiro, E., and N.P. Roos, "Retired and Employed Elderly Persons: Their Utilization of Health Care Services," *The Gerontologist* 22 (1982):187–193.

Skogland, J., "Job Deprivation in Retirement: Anticipated and Experienced Feelings," *Research on Aging* 1 (1979):481–493.

Soumerai, S.B., and J. Avorn, "Perceived Health, Life Satisfaction, and Activity in Urban Elderly: A Controlled Study of the Impact of Part-Time Work," *Journal of Gerontology* 38 (1983):356–362.

Stokes, R.G., and G.L. Maddox, "Some Social Factors on Retirement Adaptation," *Journal of Gerontology* 22 (1967):329–333.

Streib, G.F., and C.J. Schneider, *Retirement in American Society: Impact and Process* (Ithaca, N.Y.: Cornell University Press, 1971).

Thompson, G.B., "Work Versus Leisure Roles: An Investigation of Morale Among Employed and Retired Men," *Journal of Gerontology* 28 (1973): 339–344.

Thompson, W.E., G.F. Streib, and J. Kosa, "The Effect of Retirement on Personal Adjustment: A Panel Analysis," *Journal of Gerontology* 15 (1960): 165–169.

Wan, T.T.H., *Stressful Life Events, Social-Support Networks, and Gerontological Health* (Lexington, Mass.: Lexington Books, 1982).

Wan, T.T.H., B.G. Odell, and D.T. Lewis, *Promoting the Well-Being of the Elderly: A Community Diagnosis* (N.Y.: Haworth Press, 1982).

Weiner, A.I., and S.L. Hunt, "Retirees' Perceptions of Work and Leisure Meanings," *The Gerontologist* 21 (1981):444–446.

Young, M., B. Benjamin, and C. Wallis, "The Mortality of Widowers," *The Lancet* 2 (1963):454–456.

Index

Activity. *See* Participation, social
Adaptive process, phases of, 3–6
Adjustment phase of adaptation, 3, 5, 6
Age: differential in mortality, 67; frailty status and, 119; or retirement, patterns in, 9–10, 136, 148; of retirement, switching behavior and, 12–14; role losses, health consequences of, 37; role losses, social participation effects, 94–103; widowhood and, 18, 94–103
Aging: health promotion and process of, 37, 40; -related services, 129
AID analysis, 111–18
Analysis. *See* Methodology
Andersen, R., 112
Anderson, O.W., 112
Arens, D.A., 53
Atchley, R.C., 53, 75, 77, 85, 132, 154
Automatic Interaction Detector (AID) analysis, 111–18

Baker, E.L., 112
Benefits: pension, 50; social security, 15, 50, 51, 133
Berardo, F.M., 53
Bereavement. *See* Widowhood
Bernard, J., 77, 87
Bias in longitudinal studies of role loss, 67
Blacks: economic consequences of retirement for, 51; remarriage among, 157. *See also* Ethnicity; Race

California Senior Survey, 163
Campbell, R.T., 81
Care: need for, frailty and, 119–21, 128, 129, 179; need for, measuring, 109–10; "wellness," 129. *See also* Health services utilization; Planning for health and social well-being
Casscells, W., 29, 133
Cassel, J., 28
Change in retirement attitudes, 77, 81, 85, 86, 127–28
Chronic health conditions, 38–40
Clayton, P.J., 30, 52, 156, 157
Compulsory retirement, 142, 143–44, 149
Concomitance of role losses, 18, 31, 49, 54–55, 61, 103
Consumer Expenditure Survey, 143
Continuity model of well-being, 3–6, 86, 103, 127–29
Convergence in retirement attitudes in couples, 77, 78, 85–86
Coping: depression and, 170; phase of adaptation, 3, 5; resources, 68. *See also* Health service utilization; Participation, social; Retirement attitudes
Cornell Study of Occupational Retirement, 153
Coronary mortality, retirement and, 133
Couples, retirement attitudes of, 75–88
Cumulative effect of role losses, 18, 31, 49, 54–55, 61, 103

Depression, 170, 174–75

Deteriorative life changes, 91–103; defined, 92–93; social participation and, 91, 94–103, 106
Diagnostic Related Groupings, 110
Disability, physical, 9, 134, 148–49
Dissatisfaction with current activities: health status and, 112, 113, 114; social well-being and, 116, 117, 119. *See also* Participation, social
Doran, A., 28, 144
Duke Center for the Study of Aging and Human Development, 165
Duke Longitudinal Study, 31
Duke Second Longitudinal Study, 29, 147
Duke Work and Retirement Study, 29, 147

Earning test, social security, 51
Economic status: in retirement, 9, 50–51, 54, 142, 147, 153; in retirement, attitude and, 83–85; in retirement, switching behavior and, 12–14; as social participation predictor, 104; widowhood, effect on, 18, 21, 22–23, 53, 154, 161. *See also* Income
Education: level, retirement patterns and, 9–10; preretirement, 106
Ekerdt, D.J., 29, 133, 134, 135, 136
Elwell, F., 30, 91
Employment: attitudes toward, retirement attitudes and, 136–39, 150–51; hours worked, 148; impact on health, 151; opportunity for, 129, 142; prestige of, 151–52; service, 139
Ethnicity, widowhood and, 156, 160, 163
Exogenous variables. *See* Methodology
Expectations, retirement, 138, 150–51

Family, role losses and: social and economic support of, 52–53, 154, 161; social participation with, 90, 91, 93, 94–103
Females. *See* Sex differences
Ferraro, K.F., 52, 53, 158–59, 171
Financial assistance to children, widowhood and, 161
Financial planning programs, 124

Formal participation, 92, 96–103, 104, 105
Frailty status, 119–24; identifying, 109, 111; need for care and, 128, 129, 179; physician service utilization and, 121, 122; validation of classification of, 119–21
Friendship networks, 52, 90. *See also* Participation, social

Gender. *See* Sex differences
Gerontological health, components and determinants of, 3
Gerontological research, major concerns in, 1
Gianturco, D.T., 18, 30, 157, 159
Glamser, F.D., 52, 137
Gonzalez, E.R., 29, 137
Goudy, W.J., 76, 138, 139

Happiness: income and, 165; indicators of, 22; perceptions about, 56–58
Harris Study, 53
Haurin, R.J., 53, 162
Haynes, S.G., 29, 140–41
Health consequences of major role losses, 27–47, 165–67; conclusions about, 38–40; methodology of study, 31–34; related research on, 28–31; results of study, 34–38; retirement, 28–29, 31, 36–40, 128–29, 134–35, 144, 147, 165; retirement, patterns in, 7, 9, 12–14; widowhood, 19–22, 30–31, 36–40, 156–60, 167
Health service utilization, 37, 109–11, 121, 122, 150, 176–77
Health status: components and determinants of, 3; definition of, 110; employment, impact on, 151; life style and, 40, 127; perceptions of, 134, 150, 170, 171, 174, 175, 176–78; as predictor of health service use, 109–10; preventive care, 124, 129; prior levels, 112–14, 128; profiles of persons experiencing poor, 112–14; sociodemographic variables, effect of, 174. *See also* Mental health; Physical health

Heart attack, fatal, retirement and, 137
Heyman, D.K., 18, 30, 159
Hospital utilization rates, 176–77. *See also* Health service utilization
Husband, retirement attitudes of, 76–87

Impairment, retirement and, 9, 134, 148–49
Incentives for health maintenance, 124
Income: frailty and family, 121, 123; happiness and, 165; health consequences of role losses and, 37; in retirement, 50–51, 142, 147; in retirement, attitude and, 83–85; social well-being level and, 63, 116–19; of widowed, 18, 22, 53, 154, 161
Index: of physical health, 111–15; of social well-being, 111, 114–19
Inflation, impact of, ·50. *See also* Economic status; Income
Informal participation, 92, 96–103, 104, 105
Institutionalization, self-reported health status and, 171
Interaction. *See* Participation, social
Intervention strategies, 40, 68, 127
Interviews, retirement attitude study, 78–79

Jobs. *See* Employment; Retirement
Joreskog, K.G., 33, 81

Karn, V., 54, 143
Kerckhoff, A.C., 76–77, 85, 86
Kin network. *See* Family

Latency effect, 67, 127
Latent variables. *See* Methodology
Leisure: concepts, 153; retirement and, 133, 146–47. *See also* Participation, social
Life satisfaction: intervention strategies for, 68; perceptions about, 56–58; religiosity and, 173
Life Satisfaction Index, 169
Life style, establishment of healthy, 40, 127. *See also* Participation, social
Linear Structural Relationships (LISREL) model: poor physical

health estimation, 33–34, 35, 36, 38, 39; retirement attitudes estimation, 79–86; social well-being estimation, 56, 58, 60–63, 65–66, 67
Lipman, A., 76, 77, 85
LISREL model. *See* Linear Structural Relationships (LISREL) model
Livierators, B., 112
Living arrangements of widowed, 154–55, 163
Logistic regression analysis of retirement, 9–14
Longitudinal Retirement History Survey (LRHS), 2, 6; health and role losses study, 29, 31–32, 38, 145, 167; retirement attitudes study, 77–78; retirement patterns study, 8, 12; social and economic well-being study, 55, 56–58; social participation study, 91–92; targeting data from, 111–12; widowhood studies, 18–19, 161
Lopata, H.Z., 18, 52, 159
LRHS. *See* Longitudinal Retirement History Survey (LRHS)

Maddison, D., 30, 159–60
Males, social participation of older, 89–108. *See also* Sex differences
Maltbie-Crannell, A.D., 30, 91
Mandatory retirement, 142, 143–144, 149
Marital status. *See* Widowhood
Martin, J., 28, 144
Measurement: of health consequences of role losses, 32–33; of retirement attitudes, 79; of social well-being, 55. *See also* Methodology
Mental health: depression and morale, 142–43, 152, 160, 170, 174–75; life events and, 168; physical health and, 178; role losses and, 165–66; self-ratings, 169; status, 170
Methodology: in health and role losses study, 31–34; in planning for health and social well-being, 111–12; in retirement attitudes study, 77–81; in retirement patterns study, 8–9; in social and economic consequences of role losses study, 55–56, 57; in social

Methodology *(continued)*
  participation studies, 91–94; in
  widowhood study, 18–19
Migration: motivating factors, 168;
  to resorts, 143; types of, 176
Military officers, retirement of, 144
Models: of continuity of well-being,
  3–6, 86, 103, 127–29; generic, for
  explaining poor physical health,
  33–34, 40, 47, 73; generic, for
  explaining poor social well-being,
  56, 57, 59, 63; LISREL, poor
  physical health estimation,
  33–34, 35, 38, 39; LISREL,
  retirement attitudes estimation
  by, 79–86; LISREL, social well-
  being estimation, 56, 58, 60–63,
  65–66, 67
Morale: measuring, 174–75; of older
  working women, 142–43; in
  retirement, 152; in widowhood,
  160
Morbidity: self-reported, social rank
  and, 175–76; in widowhood, 162
Morgan, J.A., 112
Morrison, M.H., 50
Mortality: age and sex differential
  in, 67; relocation of elderly and,
  172; retirement, impact on, 133,
  137, 140–41, 167; self-rated
  health as predictor of, 174;
  sociodemographic variables,
  influence on, 162; of widowers,
  162–63, 164, 167
Mott, F.L., 53, 162
Mourning process, 17, 30, 164. *See
  also* Widowhood
Multiple Classification Analysis,
  93–94, 99, 112, 121, 122, 123
Mutran, E., 81, 158–59

National Longitudinal Survey, 29,
  140, 147, 148
Need for care: frailty status and,
  119–21, 128, 129, 179;
  measuring, 109–10
Norms of health services use, 110

Occupation. *See* Employment
Ohio Longitudinal Study, 29, 147
Outcome phase of adaptation, 3, 5, 6

Palmore, E.B., 29, 31, 76, 90, 147,
  148, 165–66

Panel Study of Income Dynamics,
  29, 147
Parents, support of, 52–53, 154, 161.
  See also Family
Parkes, C.M., 30, 162, 163
Partial retirement, 146
Participation, social: formal and
  informal, 92, 96–103, 104, 105; of
  older males, methodology of
  study, 91–94; of older males,
  results of study, 94–103, 106; of
  older males, roles losses and,
  89–108; perspective on, 90–91;
  planning for, 124; predictors of,
  104; in preretirement, 91, 93,
  103, 104, 106, 128; retirement
  and, 94–106, 147; widowhood
  and, 94–106, 158
Pension benefits, 50
Perceptions: of health status, 134,
  150, 170, 171, 174, 175, 176–78;
  about life satisfaction and
  happiness, 56–58; of social well-
  being, 59, 61, 63, 67, 114–19, 127
Philadelphia Geriatric Center Morale
  Scale, 169, 175
Physical health: defined, 32; generic
  model explaining poor, 33–34, 40,
  47, 73; index of, 111–15; LISREL
  model estimation of poor, 33–34,
  35, 36, 38, 39; measurement
  model of, 3, 4; mental health
  effect on, 178; prior level, 127;
  structural relationship between
  social well-being and, 63–67. *See
  also* Health status
Physician services, utilization of,
  109–111, 176–77; defining level
  of, 110–11; frailty and, 121, 122;
  health care outcomes and, 37
Planning for health and social well-
  being, 109–25; conclusions from
  study, 121–24; methodology of
  study, 111–12; related research,
  109–11; results of study, 112–21
Planning for retirement, 138
Policy, social, 105–6, 129
Preconditioned phase of adaptation,
  3, 5
Predictor trees for AID analysis,
  112–19
Preretirement: participatory life style
  in, 91, 93, 103, 104, 106, 128;
  preventive health behavior in,

124; promotion of well-being in, 68; retirement attitudes in, 153
Preventive health care, 124, 129
Psychological status. *See also* Mental health

Race: frailty status and, 119-21; remarriage and, 157; retirement and, economic consequences of, 51
Recency effect, 37, 38, 40, 67, 102, 103, 104, 120-123, 127
Regression analysis. *See* Logistic regression analysis
Religiosity, effect of, 173
Relocation of elderly, 167, 172
Remarriage: probability of, 19, 157; social participation and, 99-102, 104
Research: annotated bibliography on, 131-79; major concerns of gerontological, 1; on planning for health and social well-being, 109-11; questions on retirement attitudes, 77; on retirement process, 7-8; on social and economic consequences of role losses, 50-55; on widowhood, 17-18
Resorts, migration to, 143
Retirement: annotated bibliography on, 132-53, 165-79; concern with effects, 1; concomitant with widowhood, 18, 31, 49, 54-55, 61, 103; defined, 28; early, 165; friendships and, effect on, 90; health consequences of, 28-29, 31, 36-40, 128-29, 144, 165; leisure and, 133, 146-47; logistic regression of conditional probability of, 9-10, 11; mandatory, 142, 143-44, 149; morale in, 152; mortality rates and, 133, 137, 140-41, 167; partial, 146; as process, 8; social and economic consequences of, 50-52, 54, 55, 60, 61-62, 63, 65-67; social participation and, 94-106, 147; status, long-term influence of, 105
Retirement attitudes: conclusions from study, 86-87; of couples, 75-88; employment attitudes and, 136-39, 150-51;

expectations, 138, 150-51; of individuals, 75-76; methodology of study, 77-81; occupational prestige and, 151-52; research questions on, 77; results of study, 81-86; retirement status and, 82-83, 85; sociodemographic factors in, 132; stability in, 77, 81, 85, 86, 127-28
Retirement patterns, 7-17; age, 9-10, 136, 148; measuring, 7-8; methodology in study, 8-9; related research on, 7-8; results of study, 9-14; switching behavior, 10-14, 51
Role losses: cumulative effects, 18, 31, 49, 54-55, 61, 103; health consequences of, 27-47, 128-29, 165-67; key issues in, 1-2; social and economic consequences of, 49-73; social participation of older males and, 89-108; theoretical model of gerontological health and, 3-6; timing of, 6, 59-61, 67. *See also* Retirement; Widowhood
Role transitional phase of adaptation, 3, 5, 6
Rubin, L.B., 77

Schneider, C.J., 75
Self-employment, 140, 146
Self-perception. *See* Perception
Senior citizen activities, 129. *See also* Participation, social
Services: aging-related, 129; focus of, 128; health, utilization, 37, 109-11, 121, 122, 150, 176-77. *See also* Planning for health and social well-being
Sex differences: frailty status and, 119; intervention strategies and, 127; in mortality, 67; retirement, attitudes of couples, 75-88; retirement, patterns and, 15; retirement, switching behavior in, 12; role differentiation by, 76; role losses, health consequences of, 34-38, 39, 144; role losses, social participation and, 91, 105; self-reported health and, 171; social well-being and, 56, 58-62, 127; social well-being and, structural relationship between

Sex differences *(continued)*
  physical health and, 63–67;
  widowhood and, 18, 19, 157
Smedby, B., 112
Social networks for widowed, 52–54
Social participation. *See*
  Participation, social
Social rank: mortality during
  retirement and, 140–41; self-
  reported morbidity and, 175–76
Social Security Administration, 92;
  Retirement History Study
  Sample, 138, 147
Social security benefits, 15, 50, 51,
  133
Social well-being: index of, 111,
  114–19; measurement of, 3, 4,
  55, 56, 57; perception of, 59, 61,
  63, 67, 114–19, 127; prior levels,
  as preconditioned factors, 128;
  profiles of persons perceiving
  negative, 114–19; retirement and,
  52; role losses and, 54–55, 58–62;
  structural relationship between
  physical and, 63–67
Socioeconomic status: health and,
  40, 147; indicators of, 22;
  retirement and, 136; social
  participation and, 91, 93, 106;
  widowhood and, 21, 22–23
Somatic complaints, 135
Sonquist, J.N., 112
Sorbom, D., 33, 79
Stability in retirement attitudes, 77,
  81, 85, 86, 127–28
Streib, G.F., 75, 153
Stress: psychological symptoms of,
  168–69; widowhood and, 154. *See
  also* Role losses
Structural relationship between
  physical and social well-being,
  63–67
Suicide rate of widowed, 155
Survey of Low-Income Aged and
  Disabled, 158
Switched retirement status, 10–14,
  51

Targeting approach, 109–25
Timing of role losses, 6, 59–61, 67

Unemployment, 172–73. *See also*
  Retirement

Validation of frailty classification,
  119–21
Variables. *See* Methodology
Veterans Administration Normative
  Aging Study, 29, 134, 135, 136
Viola, A., 30, 159–60

Wages, impairment and, 134
Wan, T.T.H., 17, 29, 54, 112, 167,
  179
Well-being of elderly: components
  and determinants of, 3;
  continuity model of, 3–6, 86,
  103, 127–29. *See also* Health
  status; Social well-being
"Wellness care," 129
Wheaton, B., 79
Widowhood, 17–25; analysis of data
  on, 19–23; annotated bibliography
  on, 154–67; concomitant with
  retirement, 31, 54–55, 61, 103;
  ethnicity and, 156, 160, 163;
  friendships and, effect on, 90;
  health consequences of, 19–22,
  30–31, 36–40, 156–60, 167; kin
  relations, impact on, 52–53, 90,
  161; living arrangements during,
  154–55, 163; methodology of
  study, 18–19; morale in, 160;
  mortality in, 162, 164, 167;
  related research on, 17–18; sex
  differences in, 18, 19, 157; social
  and economic consequences of,
  18, 22, 52–54, 154, 161; social
  participation and, 94–106, 158;
  social psychological status in,
  154–55; suicide rates, 155
Wives, retirement attitudes of,
  76–87
Work. *See* Employment; Retirement
World Health Organization, 110

Young, M., 30, 164

Zung Self-Rating Depression Scale,
  175

About the Author

Thomas T. H. Wan is professor of health administration and director of the Doctoral Program in Health Administrative Sciences at the Medical College of Virginia, Virginia Commonwealth University. He is a medical sociologist who has been on the faculties of the University of Maryland Baltimore County and Cornell University, and he has also served as a Senior Research Fellow of the National Center for Health Services Research. Dr. Wan did his undergraduate work at Tunghai University in Taiwan and received his M.A. (1968) and Ph.D. (1970) in sociology from the University of Georgia; he also received an M.H.S. degree from the Johns Hopkins University School of Hygiene and Public Health (1971), where he was an NIH postdoctoral fellow.

Dr. Wan is a member of many professional societies and a fellow of the Gerontological Society of America. He serves as a member of the Executive Council of the Association for the Social Sciences in Health. He has also served as a consultant to the National Center for Health Services Research. His current research focuses on the determinants and consequences of institutionalization, evaluation of long-term care programs, and epidemiology of falls. As a health services researcher, he has published numerous articles and books in the health care field.